the
GINSENGS

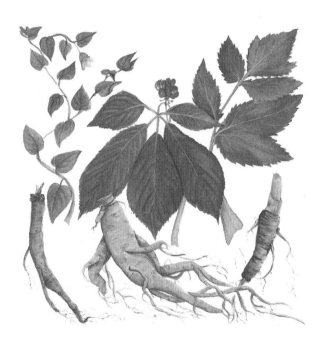

the
GINSENGS
A USER'S GUIDE

Christopher Hobbs, L.Ac.

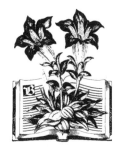

BOTANICA PRESS

This book is printed on recycled paper

Look for these books by Christopher Hobbs –
available from Botanica Press:

The Herbs and Health Series:
Echinacea! The Immune Herb
Foundations of Health
Ginkgo, Elixir of Youth
Handbook for Herbal Healing
Kombucha, Manchurian Tea Mushroom
Medicinal Mushrooms
Milk Thistle, The Liver Herb
Natural Liver Therapy
Usnea, Herbal Antibiotic
Valerian, The Relaxing and Sleep Herb
Vitex, The Women's Herb

NEW!
Christopher Hobbs' Herbal Prescriber (herbs on disk)

BOTANICA PRESS, 10226 Empire Grade, Santa Cruz, CA 95060

Table of Contents

the Ginsengs:
A User's Guide

By Christopher Hobbs

———

Introduction

As one of the most popular human remedies of all time, the ancient herb ginseng is surprisingly little-understood by today's modern herb user. If you are among these users and are confused by the hype or hoopla, don't feel alone—many herbalists and scientists who study medicinal plants as their life's work are also confused about ginseng. Since there are few, if any, practical guides to the many uses and benefits of ginseng, we wrote this book to make the world's literature and experience about ginseng more accessible. As an herbalist with nearly thirty years of experience, I have encountered many people who were misinformed about this ancient herb. While traveling and lecturing in North America, Australia, and Europe, I find that the most common questions people ask about herbs concern ginseng. Such questions as these are indicative:

- ➤ *Does ginseng prolong life and increase energy?*
- ➤ *Is ginseng just for men and not women?*
- ➤ *Can ginseng help increase sexual energy? Is it an aphrodisiac?*
- ➤ *What is the best kind of ginseng?*
- ➤ *What is the difference between Siberian, red, white, and American ginsengs? Which is best?*
- ➤ *Is ginseng good for bodybuilders, and does it help increase muscle mass?*
- ➤ *Can ginseng help relieve the distressing symptoms of hangovers?*
- ➤ *How does one take ginseng and for how long?*
- ➤ *What are the best kinds of products available?*
- ➤ *How many types of ginseng are there and how are they used?*

We hope to clearly answer these questions and more. In these pages we have included concise summaries of the historical record of a number of medicinal plants known as ginseng, as well as a short review of the scientific studies that have been performed on many of them, especially focusing on true ginseng, *Panax ginseng* C.A. Meyer, and eleuthero or Siberian ginseng, *Eleutherococcus senticosus* (Rupr. Et Maxim.) Maxim. We have included relevant clinical reports from practitioners who use ginseng products, plus useful information on how to make ginseng extracts at home and how to use them. Finally, we have included summaries of eight kinds of traditional herbs often called ginseng in Traditional Chinese Medicine (TCM), concise tables that compare and contrast the uses at a glance, as well as a "prescriber" of symptoms and syndromes, and an indication of which ginseng is best for each.

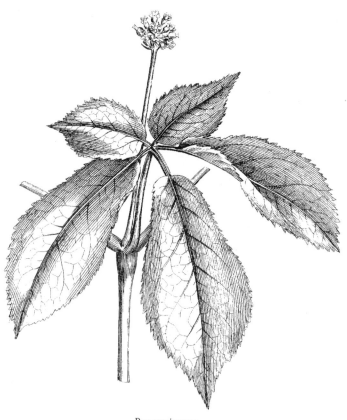

Panax ginseng
from *Histoire Naturelle des Végétaux* by E. Spach, 1846

PART ONE
What is Ginseng?

Ginseng is surrounded by controversy. In Asia, the herb is a cultural jewel and a daily necessity for millions. In the west, it is considered a useful energy-promoting herb at best and is viewed with extreme skepticism by western scientists, who often conclude that ginseng is a cultural fraud. Table 1 compares both sides of some controversial issues surrounding ginseng.

TABLE 1: AN HONEST EVALUATION OF GINSENG AT A GLANCE

Positive Benefits	Possible Drawbacks
3-5,000 years of use by millions; an important herb in one of the most eloquent and widely-used medical systems in the world (Traditional Chinese Medicine)	Cultural acceptance might border on superstition
Hundreds of laboratory experiments	Very few controlled human studies
Active constituents are fairly stable; high-quality ginseng is available	Many products contain inferior quality herb, and unstandardized products vary in content of active constituents
Contains antioxidants	Many common foods have much higher antioxidant activity

THE POPULARITY OF GINSENG

Today herbal medicine is making a rapid comeback in developed countries around the world. In many countries, like China, India, and South America, herbal medicine is commonly used by people as a primary means of staying healthy. It is an important aid for alleviating the symptoms of disease and working with the body's innate healing powers to rid itself of disease and reestablish health.

All herbs are not unquestionably safe under every circumstance, and no responsible person trained in herbal medicine would say that they are, but most are far safer than highly-purified and manufactured modern drugs, and their use is much easier on our environment. Their use does not pollute our air and water, as does the manufacture of synthetic drugs. Many leading practitioners of medicine are convinced there is a need and place for both in the modern health practice.

Today, many doctors and other health practitioners are called upon to work with patients who have symptoms difficult to define and even more difficult to diagnose. Some examples are chronic fatigue, generalized aches and pains, depression, overweight, confusion, nervousness, anxiety, and dizziness. Many doctors can only prescribe aspirin, antidepressives, sleeping pills, and sedatives, or finally, when these don't work, a psychiatric evaluation. But to the people who have these symptoms, it is not "all in their head;" their symptoms are only too real. Although we might not like to think so, perhaps many of these symptoms can be related to the stresses of modern life and just plain poor health habits. A group of health researchers and practitioners who run a health retreat in the Bahamas (Popov et al, 1974) have summed up the problem well:

"The men and women exposed to the stress of modern life, contaminated and polluted surroundings, inadequate nutrition, constant noise and nervous tension, suffer from many syndromes undetectable by physical examinations or laboratory tests. The most frequent complaints are tiredness, sleeplessness, bad digestion, loss of memory, obesity, impotence, bad temper and looks, flabby flesh and many other signs for which the physician—who too often has the same sufferings—is unable to do anything."

What is the answer? In my experience, many symptoms can be alleviated by learning and practicing simple health habits. These include proper nutrition, suitable for our *individual* needs, proper breathing, exercise, the creation and practice of good relationships, and adequate rest. Learning to relax with the help of meditation, prayer, mindfulness, stretching, yoga, tai qi, and other tools are also important. See the Appendix for a few suggestions of tapes and books that can help. When people would ask my revered teacher, Paul C. Bragg, what he had for specific ailments or symptoms such as arthritis, he would always answer that he had no specifics—only a total program for health!

However, this is not to say that there are no herbs or remedies in nature's medicine chest that cannot help. Throughout history, we have sought ease from our suffering as well as an improvement in our energy and performance with herbal remedies.

As one of the oldest and most revered herbs in human history, ginseng, or *Panax ginseng* C.A. Meyer, as the botanists have dubbed it, is experiencing an unprecedented increase in popularity throughout

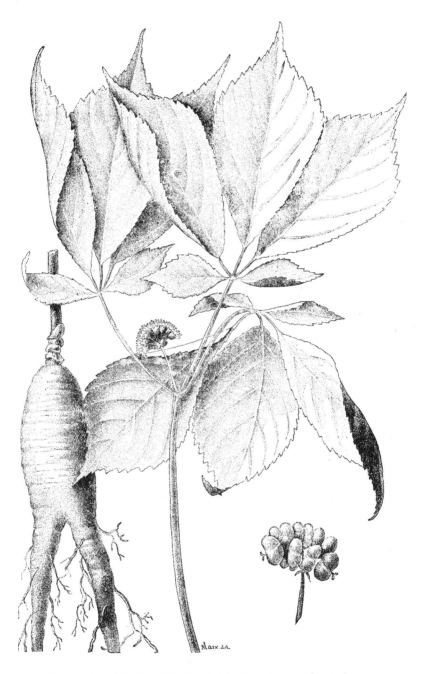

Panax quinquefolius from *The Report of the Commissioner of Agriculture*
by the Department of Agriculture, 1884

Asia, North America, Europe, Australia, New Zealand, and other countries. As an example of ginseng's increasing popularity, in the United States all ginseng sales were estimated to have nearly tripled to 10.8 million dollars during the year ending August 31, 1992 (Deveny, 1992). Over 90% of the total crop is exported to Asian buyers (Fryer, 1995). Ginsana, a nationally-advertised ginseng product "standardized," or adjusted, to a consistent level of compounds that are thought to be responsible for the herb's activity, accounted for about 92% of the sales.

Because of the amazing increase in popularity, pressures on wild ginseng, which has become nearly extinct in Asia because of centuries of overharvesting, have dramatically increased in the last ten years in North America as well. This has led to decreases in populations throughout its natural range, which is from Quebec, Ontario, and Manitoba in the north down through parts of northern Florida, Alabama, Louisiana, and Oklahoma.

It is only natural, then, that cultivation of such a popular crop would also dramatically increase, and it has—and then some! The *Wall Street Journal* recently reported that the world's largest ginseng grower, Chai-Na-Ta Corporation, a British Columbia company, recently had sales of 19.1 million dollars US in the year ending Nov. 30, 1994 (*WSJ*, Business Brief, Thu, Nov 30, 1995). The company reported a record harvest of 483,000 pounds of ginseng root, 52% more than the previous year.

Traditionally, much of the cultivated American ginseng is grown in Wisconsin because of the cool, moist summers and freezing winters that ginseng prefers. The farms were pioneered by German-Americans in the early 1900s, and today newcomers are viewed with suspicion, some farmers even burning excess seed to avoid competition (Ingersoll, 1992). In the early days of cultivation, farmers brought wild roots in from the woods and grew the plants under shade cloth, finding that ginseng does not grow well in direct sunlight.

Today, ginseng dealers from Asia, especially Hong Kong, can be seen cruising down Wisconsin and, increasingly, Canadian highways in the late fall, cellular phone in hand, "searching for their roots." It's a colorful sight and one that seems incongruous, except for the shared passion for ginseng. The buying frenzy continues for nearly three months, while growers and dealers alike work eighteen hour days. The roots, which are kiln-dried through the crisp autumn days and frigid starry nights, are airshipped to Hong Kong for distribution to centers throughout Asia. Though fortunes can be made on ginseng, it is a risky business. Throughout the 4-5 years of growth, ginseng roots are susceptible to fungus attack that can turn them into mush almost overnight. It is estimated to take 5-10 years to break even on an initial investment of capital to start a ginseng farm.

Canadian ginseng is very much up-and-coming these days. From 1990 through 1994, production is estimated to have grown about 325%, and by 1996, Canada's harvest will be second only to China in world production (Turner, 1995). The center of Canada's agricultural efforts is focused in British Columbia, where production is estimated by government sources to nearly triple in the next four years.

In China, the production of ginseng is probably over 5,000 tons. In parts of rural China, almost every small growing cooperative has its ginseng patch (Parks, 1983). Before the 1960s, the common person in China could not often afford ginseng. In fact, only about 10% of the population could formerly obtain it on a regular basis (Hu, 1976). This has mostly changed today with widespread cultivation and rising prosperity in China. Since today many Chinese people (the population of China is 1.2 billion) start taking ginseng by age 40 to slow aging and prevent illness, it is obvious that the market for this herb is nothing short of phenomenal. The Chinese believe that ginseng can fight cancer, slow aging, protect one against heart attack and other sudden illnesses, strengthen digestion, and reduce high blood pressure, among numerous other benefits (Parks, 1983). In China, Ginseng is found in every imaginable form—capsules, tablets, teas, candy wines, chewing gum, and especially in Chinese cuisine. A famous chef in Changchun, the capital of Jilin province from where half of China's ginseng comes, has even written a cookbook devoted solely to ginseng cuisine.

The best ginseng in China is affordable only by the elite and is said to be literally "worth its weight in gold." This top grade is called "heaven grade," lesser quality roots being know as "earth grade" and "man grade." Although many people think of ginseng as an aphrodisiac, it is not often considered so in Chinese medicine. A researcher from the Jilin Special Products Institute in China said that ginseng does not ". . . lead you to do things that you would not do anyway." another colleague added that ginsengs ". . . just strengthen you to do what is normal." Ginseng is thought to help men overcome sexual imbalances such as impotence, however.

THE HISTORY AND TRADITION OF GINSENG

Ginseng (*Panax ginseng*) is one of the oldest and almost certainly among the most famous herbs in world history. It has been used in China for thousands of years, usually combined with other herbs, to restore vital energy, especially in the elderly and people weakened by illness. It is a main ingredient in hundreds of formulas in Traditional Chinese Medicine (TCM), a medical system utilized by perhaps half of the world's population.

Some authors believe ginseng has been in continuous use in China for over 4,000 years (Duke, 1989). Other reports place the introduction of the herb at about 2,000 years ago or less. Indeed, the origins of the use of ginseng are probably lost in the obscure mists of time. Chinese scholars, though, are very clear that the first mention of the herb in a book of medicinal plant use or materia medica (*Ben Cao* or *Pen T'sao*) is in the *Classic of the Materia Medica* from the mythical "Divine Husbandman" (shen nung or shen nong) (Hu, 1977). The Divine Husbandman is a legendary figure, supposedly flourishing in the 28th Century B.C., who is said to have introduced agriculture and animal husbandry. He is also the patron of herbal medicine. The book is thought to be compiled by a group of writers from the Han period (B.C. 202-A.D. 221), but derived from much earlier writings. It is still considered to be of the highest authority by Chinese herbalists. By tradition, the drugs mentioned (252 botanical entries) in the work are still kept in modern herbal shops under the same ancient names (Bretschneider, 1895). A revision of the work by Tao Hung-Ching (AD 452-536) includes the passage from which this quote is taken:

> *It grows in the gorges of the mountains. It is used for repairing the five viscera, quieting the spirit, curbing the emotions, stopping agitation, removing noxious influences, brightening the eyes, enlightening the mind and increasing wisdom. Continuous use leads one to longevity with light weight* (Hu, 1977).

Other ancient Chinese legends hold that the use of ginseng was brought by the great Chinese philosopher, Lao Tzu (604 B.C.), or Confucius, who is said to have given a discourse on the herb about 2,500 years ago (Duke, 1989).

According to Chinese scholars and scientists the *Ben cao gang mu* (or simply *Ben cao* or *Pen T'sao*), the greatest compilation of Chinese medicinal plants ever written (in 1590 by Li Shi-Zhen), describes five "shens" or medicinal roots. These five herbal remedies are said to positively affect the 5 major internal organs (Bretschneider, 1895; Smith & Stuart, 1973).

➤ Ren shen or true ginseng (*Panax ginseng*) which strengthens the Spleen (the organ system that assimilates and digests our food in Chinese medicine)

➤ Sha shen or white ginseng (*Adenophora polymorpha* Ledeb.) which is considered strengthening to the lungs

➤ Xuan shen or black ginseng (*Scrophularia oldhami* Oliv.) which supports the Kidneys and adrenals

➤ Dan shen or red ginseng (*Salvia miltiorrhiza* Bunge), which is strengthening to the heart; (not to be confused with steamed *Panax ginseng*, also called red ginseng)

➤ Mou shen or purple ginseng (*Polygonum bistorta* L.) which acts on the liver

Of the five, true ginseng is considered the most valuable and potent for lengthening life and promoting vitality. It is significant that true ginseng mainly supports digestive function, because Chinese herbalists, like western herbalists, consider that the digestive system is at the center of all of the other body systems, and of all of them, it is the most responsible for supplying Qi (pronounced "chee"), or vitality, to the entire body. It is the true "foundation of health."

Although ginseng is one of the most popular herbs in trade worldwide, by itself it is rarely used as a *cure* for anything. However, it does play a role in hundreds of curative herbal formulas. Ironically, that is why it is so esteemed in China and the oriental systems of medicine that have arisen in Korea, Vietnam, Japan, and elsewhere. Rather than cure a specific condition, it restores deficient Qi, or vital energy, and regulates or balances the functions of important body systems. In TCM, that makes it a "superior" medicine, because it is thought that the primary purpose of the healing arts is to restore balance and strength and empower the body to heal itself. Herbs that treat specific conditions abound in TCM, but they are considered inferior to—and are often paired with—the superior herbs that restore balance and strength. In the west, we are just beginning to embrace the concept of natural herbs and foods that can restore balance and increase vigor in more than one body system, such as the nervous system and the hormonal system. These substances are called "adaptogens." More information about adaptogens can be found in the next section.

Qi, Blood, Yin & Yang – The Components of Life

Throughout this book you will come across the terms Yin, Yang, Qi, and Blood. Blood is well-known to westerners as the fluid that carries oxygen, sugars and other nutrients, immune substances, and waste products in and out of the cells of the body. The other concepts are not well-known in the west, and it is difficult to fully understand the action and uses of the ginsengs, and Chinese medicine itself, without an understanding of these 4 concepts.

Yin and Yang are the most basic concepts not only of Chinese medicine, but in Chinese culture and life as well. In the world of cause and effect (the phenomenal world), existence is divided into pairs of opposites that balance and complement each other to create a whole. Thus, because the two halves make a whole and cannot exist without the other, when one aspect is waxing, the other is waning. For instance, when the light is increasing, darkness is decreasing; as it gets hotter, cold is decreasing. In TCM, the two "umbrella" concepts for all the pairs of opposites are called Yin and Yang. Each has its own nature and can be defined by the pairs that relate with it. For instance, Yin is associated with coldness, the feminine aspect, darkness, and inward movement, and thus nurturing. Yang is associated with heat, light, action or activity, and outward movement.

For health to occur, Yin and Yang must be in balance. In other words, there can neither be too much heat or cold, not too much activity or nourishment (catabolism versus anabolism). In western concepts, Yin and Yang might be related to matter and energy. Matter is solid and represents a denser manifestation of energy, whereas energy is active and expansive and represents matter breaking down to release energy, like wood burning to produce heat and light.

Each cell, organ and organ system, and ultimately the entire body as a harmonious association of systems must all have this Yin-Yang balance. As one of my favorite TCM teachers was fond of saying "Nothing escapes Yin-Yang Theory." In other words, everything in the universe is governed by this. This is the primary law of physics according to Chinese thinking and TCM.

According to TCM, the preservation of health and treatment of disease are accomplished by balancing pairs of opposites that are considered important to the function of the body. However, Yin and Yang balance is the concept that is often considered first and last.

The use of herbs is one of the most important ways in which we can change the Yin-

Ginseng may be ancient and esteemed, but it is also, at least in the West, greatly misunderstood and less appreciated than in the Orient, as we have previously hinted. It is also very expensive, which provides a profit motive for companies (as well as governments) to advertise its reputation and promote it as a cure-all or "panacea," which is what its Latin name (*Panax*) implies.

Yang balance of the cells, organs, and tissues, and thus restore health to the individual. Various ginsengs can promote either Yin or Yang, depending on the type, how much is taken, and under what circumstances. The specifics of this statement can be found throughout this book.

While Yin and Yang are general concepts to help organize and explain how existence in the phenomenal world might work, Yin is also associated with specific substances in the body. Thus if one's body is too metabolically active, for instance under the influence of stimulants like expresso, the Yin substances (moisture, blood, sexual hormones, etc.) can be depleted, causing one to become "dried out." In this case, we want to "tonify the Yin." If the body becomes metabolically underactive (sluggish metabolism), and there is not enough functional energy to transform stored energy, such as glucose, to heat and muscle movement, then things can become generally sluggish and cold. If our metabolism is too slow, we can become heavier and carry excess fat and phlegm, to the point of inhibiting the proper nutrition of the cells and organs in the body. In this case, there is lack of movement and release of energy—we need to "tonify the Yang."

The term Qi is generally translated to mean energy or vitality. However, in Chinese medicine, there are a number of types of Qi. This discussion is beyond the scope of this book, but the excellent books *The Web That Has No Weaver* (Kaptchuk, 1983) or *Between Heaven and Earth: A Guide to Chinese Medicine* (Korngold & Beinfield, 1991) can help eloquently explain these and other terms used in Chinese Medicine in western terms. In this book, Qi will be taken to mean vitality, mainly. Qi is the force that causes the blood to move through the vessels, the lungs to take air in and out, the body to move, the mind to think, and the immune system to ward off pathogens. In fact, in TCM, the total power of the immune system to expel disease-causing agents (the pathogens) is called the "Antipathogenic Qi." Conversely, the power or vitality of the pathogen is known as the "Pathogenic Qi." To overcome many diseases, such as colds and flu, we want to "tonify the anti-pathogenic Qi." Chinese medicine says that if our anti-pathogenic Qi is stronger than the pathogenic Qi, we will get better.

In modern societies we want all the Qi we can get! Ginseng is probably best-known for increasing the Qi of the body, and thus helping all functions of the body to work better.

The Names of Ginseng

Ginseng's name owes its origins to a German scientist, Carl Anton Meyer, who gave it a modern Latin binomial in 1842. To this day, the full scientific name is sometimes given as *Panax ginseng* C.A. Meyer. *Panax* is derived from the Greek *pan*, "all," and *akos*, "cure," meaning a cure-all or panacea (Hu, 1976).

Dr. Shiu Ying Hu, the renowned botanical scholar, formerly of Arnold Arboretum, Boston, has said that

. . . the sound gin stands for the Chinese word for "man" and seng is the equivalent of "essence" (very close in pronunciation), the substance that underlies all outward manifestations. According to a conventional Chinese belief, ginseng is the crystallization of the essence of the earth in the form of a man. It represents the vital spirit of the earth that dwells in a root. It is the manifestation of the spiritual phase of nature in material form.

The word "sang" or "seng" (short for ginseng) is commonly used by rural pickers in the Eastern United States. By comparison, the word "seng" is known by Chinese medicinal plant diggers to mean any of a number of fleshy medicinal roots. The word is usually modified by different words, depending on its source and medicinal use. Besides "jen-seng," there are "xuan-seng," "sa-seng," and "tang-seng," as well as others (Hu, 1976).

Other popular Chinese names (at least their English equivalents) include "long-life root," "divine herb," "man's health," "root of life," "queen of the orient," "promise of immortality," "wonder root," and "man plant."

GINSENG & ITS RELATIVES, BOTANICALLY SPEAKING

There are only a few kinds of true ginsengs in the botanical genus *Panax*, and there are others that are in the ginseng family, but more distantly related to ginseng botanically, such as eleuthero ("Siberian ginseng"). Certain ginsengs are not botanically related at all but affect the body functions in similar ways. These include plants in the bell-flower family (Campanulaceae) such as codonopsis (*Codonopsis pilosula* Franch.), which is also called dan shen, or sha shen (*Adenophora triphilla* DC. subsp. *aperticampanulata* Kitamura), and other species of *Adenophora,* or glehnia (*Glehnia littoralis* F. Schmidt ex Miq.) which is in the parsley family (Apiaceae). Each kind of "ginseng"—for example, red Korean *Panax ginseng*, white Chinese *Panax ginseng*, Eleuthero (Siberian ginseng), or codonopsis—has its own therapeutic character, taste, and properties; in other words, its own "energy." For an excellent account of many kinds of ginseng, the processing methods, and ginseng substitutes used in China, see Hu (1976).

Some ginsengs are strong, hot, and Yang and are particularly useful for extremely debilitated people, the very old, or people recovering from operations or severe medical conditions (red Korean ginseng). Others are milder and cooler, supporting both Yin (vital essence) and Yang (vital function) and are more appropriate for younger people experiencing stress and "burnout" (eleuthero or American ginseng). Others, such as "Brazilian ginseng" (*Pfaffia paniculata* [Mart.] Kuntze or suma) are classed inappropriately with ginseng to benefit from its superb reputation. It is best to avoid referring to these herbs as ginseng, as this only adds to the confusion about their appropriate use.

Ginseng can be a very effective herb when used properly. The main purpose of this book is to help the reader distinguish between the different kinds of ginseng and understand how each can be used in different contexts. For example, ginseng has a reputation for strengthening sexual function. There may be some truth to this, as we'll see. Yet if it works, it works primarily in people whose production of sexual hormones has begun to decline, through age or illness. Consider, on the other hand, a young man, in search of sexual prowess, who turns to ginseng. Perhaps he wants the "best," so he purchases the strongest red Korean ginseng. Yet that is the most yang, heating, and stimulating of all the ginsengs, and our young man, being healthy, may already be full of overheated yang energy. His stress may actually stem from excess energy, and what he needs for balance are more cooling, nourishing, and relaxing foods and herbs, such as reishi or eleuthero. Creating a better balance between Yin and Yang may help him improve his sexual function. Red ginseng, on the other hand, may be too overheating for his temperament. Rather than improve his sexual function, it might actually impair it.

THE SCIENCE OF GINSENG—IS IT CREDIBLE?

There is no doubt that in the realm of folk medicine and traditional medicine, ginseng is one of the most widely-used herbal remedies of all time. But what does science have to say about the effectiveness of ginseng and ginseng products? Does modern science support its use for some or all of the effects and conditions we have discussed above? This is not an easy question to answer; it depends on the point of view of the person considering the data. The main problem with the science of ginseng—at least for western scientists—is not the quantity of studies that have been performed, but the quality. If one wanted to gather together all the published clinical reports, laboratory analyses, animal studies, and human studies, the end result would be an impressive stack of papers. However, most of these studies have been performed in China and published in Chinese, which renders many of them inaccessible to western readers, though a good portion have English abstracts available in on-line databases.

In reviewing the studies that are available in English, it is evident that about 95% of them are either about testing ginseng extracts or the individual ginsenosides (considered the main active constituents) in animals, animal cell cultures, or human cell cultures to determine the pharmacological effect. How these studies translate to actual clinical efficacy and safety is yet to be seen. The clinical studies with human volunteers, for the most part, do not include a control group, or are not "blinded" to attempt to eliminate the placebo effect and the bias of the investigators and participants. The bottom line is that for one of the most popular herbs in the world, ginseng has very few modern well-designed human controlled studies to its credit. This may be because in China the placebo effect is considered an acceptable part of the overall effectiveness of an herb or remedy. It is also sometimes the case that Chinese researchers do not consider it ethical to withhold the herb in one group of sick people and give only a placebo. Herbal remedies are a very ingrained part of the Chinese culture, and after 4,000 or 5,000 years of continuous study and ancestral use, it is considered improper to question their efficacy. The Chinese ginseng researcher might ask the question, "*Why* does it work?;" while the western scientist asks, "*Does* it work?" Modern Chinese researchers are aware, however, that for westerners to accept ginseng as a valuable remedy or preventative tonic, there needs to be more well-designed studies, and this is beginning to happen.

In defense of ginseng, the amazing tradition of use of the herb in millions of people, and for so long, literally millennia, must count for something. For one thing, it appears to be reasonably safe. Though any herb has potential contraindications and cautions, if used with some knowledge, ginseng is unlikely to aggravate any health condition or worsen symptoms of disease. It is very unlikely to be at all dangerous, even in overdoses.

When considering the safety and efficacy of ginseng, Traditional Chinese Medicine has very clear guidelines about who should use it and when and under what circumstances. If these guidelines are understood and followed, the user will be much more likely to experience clear beneficial results. It is difficult to accept that the use of such a massively popular herb is simply a cultural superstition—akin to mass hysteria or mass hypnosis.

There are enough scientific studies to show clearly that ginseng and ginseng extracts have pharmacological effects in animals and humans, and the evidence is mounting.

A major part of the problem of acceptance of ginseng in the West may be purely cultural. Westerners are not keen on accepting the whole concept of adaptogens, which are natural substances that can promote general health, well-being, and balance in body cells, tissues, organs, and entire systems, as well as help prevent disease. To the western mind, the whole idea smacks of quackery. Instead, we tend to think that there is a single "cause and effect" participating in every disease, and that there are very specific drugs that can alleviate symptoms or cure the disease. According to medical science, AIDS is caused by a particular virus, and the myriad of other factors that weaken the human immune system in the first place, allowing the virus to flourish, are not considered important.

The more narrow the indications for a drug, the more comfortable modern medicine is with it. And the more comfortable regulatory agencies are with it, indeed, because it is easier to control and regulate the profits from a purified and patented drug. But to the Chinese, and increasingly to more open western minds, the body is not a collection of departments that are isolated from each other. What affects one part of the body affects the whole body. Every part is interconnected—just as every living thing on earth is interconnected, and the health of one part affects the whole. In the Orient, one considers the whole, and places more emphasis on health. In the Occident, the focus is on the specific, and the emphasis is often on disease. For instance, a western doctor might make a diagnosis of arthritis and prescribe drugs, such as aspirin, to suppress inflammation and pain. A TCM doctor will likely try to determine what imbalances are present in the whole body, and support or regulate the kidneys (plus the adrenals), the digestive system, or any other system that is in need of fine-tuning. Neither western medicine nor eastern medicine is "right" or better. To create a whole medicine that treats a whole person, an understanding of both health and disease, as well an understanding of the microcosm and macrocosm, are needed to paint the entire picture. For a review of the science of ginseng, see *The Nature of the True Ginsengs* below.

Ginseng—Is it Worth the Price?

A good example of the western mindset about the value of ginseng can be found in a book on *Panax* by James Duke, Ph.D., a well-respected herbal researcher and botanist. Dr. Duke is appreciated by herbalists and scientists alike for his humor and balanced approach to writing and educating people about herbs. He has consistently supported the use of herbs and foods for healing throughout his career as a botanist with the United States Department of Agriculture (USDA). In his book *Ginseng*, he makes a comparison between ginseng and the common carrot. His contention is that because of the lack of credible controlled human studies on the efficacy of ginseng, the carrot would be a better choice for everyday use as an adaptogenic and preventative substance. He cites research about the use of carrots as a cancer protector, antioxidant, and body regulator and emphasizes the great difference in price between the two. Even the finest organic carrots go for less than a dollar a pound and good wild ginseng for over $300, though naturally-cultivated roots can be had for under $60. This seems like a good argument—carrots *are* excellent protectors and a very healthy food indeed. And they are a very ancient food, though written records don't go back as far as ginseng. But an average effective dose of ginseng is approximately 1-9 grams of dry root and the carrot ten to thirty times that amount or more. Ginseng takes an average of three to six years to develop with much difficulty in cultivation to bring it to optimum size and strength, and a carrot takes six months. Considering this, the price difference seems more reasonable.

To the Chinese, it would be difficult to put a price on a cultural legacy of 5,000 years of revered human use. Ginseng is an integral part of a fantastic art-form and scientific endeavor called Traditional Chinese Medicine worked out by millions of people. TCM can be considered one of the most subtle, yet elegant and powerful systems of health and disease ever devised. It has sprung up from the very stuff of the earth from which we came. It looks at the human relationship with regard to the seasons, the elements, the diet, and the emotions as healing and disease-promoting influences.

In the following sections we will explore more of the folklore and science of ginseng and ginseng-like plants. Whether you ultimately choose carrots or ginseng as your "tonic of choice" is a personal decision, but we hope to provide a clear picture of ginseng, so that your decision will be a well-informed one.

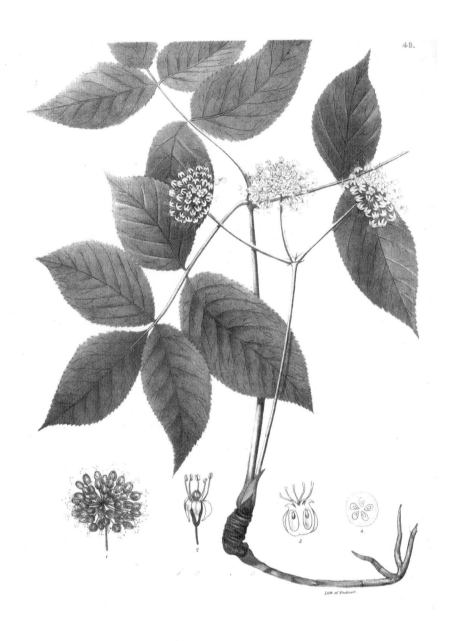

Aralia nudicaulis—"False Ginseng" or "Fool's Ginseng" has fooled many a ginseng hunter.
from *Natural History of New York* by J. Torrey, 1843

THE TYPES OF GINSENG: AN OVERVIEW

It is worthwhile to gain some clarity on the many herbs that travel under the name of ginseng. There are different varieties of true ginsengs, as well as differences in cultivation and manufacturing processes, each of which is relevant to how the herb affects the body and for which kinds of conditions it is best suited. Other herbs are not true ginsengs at all but are classified functionally in TCM with the ginsengs, because they have similar effects. True ginsengs are considered to be only those herbs in the genus *Panax* from the Ginseng family, Araliaceae, by western science as well as western herbalists. This is in contrast to Chinese herbalists who often do not draw distinctions between herbs based on botanical characteristics alone, but on other properties such as taste, temperature, and actions in the body.

A plant family, which is a natural group with very similar characteristic floral or chemical features, consists of one to many *genera* (single, *genus*), which themselves consist of one to many species. For instance the Mint family, Lamiaceae, consists of the genera *Salvia* (sages), *Rosmarinus* (rosemary), *Thymus* (thyme), and *Mentha* (the mints), among others. Within the genus *Mentha*, there are a number of familiar species, namely *Mentha spicata* L. (spearmint), *Mentha x piperita* L. (peppermint), and *Mentha pulegeum* L. (pennyroyal).

Considering the true ginsengs from the genus *Panax*, let's start with *Panax ginseng*, or Oriental ginseng. Chinese and Korean ginseng are both *Panax ginseng*. This is the most common kind of ginseng and the main ingredient of many ginseng products, especially if they originate from Asia. It is also the most commonly cultivated ginseng in the world. You can purchase *Panax ginseng* in many forms, from whole root to powders to teas to supplements that contain a guaranteed amount of ginsenosides.

The two main kinds of *Panax ginseng* are white and red. This refers not to botanical differences, but to manufacturing methods. White *Panax ginseng*, whether Chinese or Korean, is the root that has been peeled and dried. Red *Panax ginseng*, primarily Korean, has been steamed with the peel left on and then dried. This process is very effective at preserving ginseng from pests, and it also creates some chemical changes. Scientific studies confirm that red ginseng contains different ginsenosides (Chong and Oberholzer, 1988), which helps explain their different effects.

Red ginseng is the hottest and most yang of the ginsengs, which makes it the best kind for people over 40 whose hormonal "fires" have begun to cool off. It is also most appropriate for very debilitated people, and particularly inappropriate for younger (under 40), generally healthy people who are suffering from overheated conditions, often brought on by the daily use of stimulants (such as coffee and cola drinks) and a big helping of stress. Chinese researchers have also shown red ginseng to be superior in promoting good blood circulation, reducing abnormal clotting, and invigorating the elderly (Li et al, 1991).

White Asian ginseng (mainly Korean or Chinese) is a cooler ginseng and is a general-purpose ginseng useful for people who need a little energy boost. It is not as stimulating as red ginseng and is thought to strengthen the digestion and promote longevity.

The next kind of true ginseng is American ginseng, *Panax quinquefolius* L., which means "five-leafed *Panax*." This ginseng, indigenous to North America only, has an appearance similar to that of *P. ginseng*, and grows in the hardwood forests of Eastern North America, commonly occurring on cool north slopes along with sugar maple and red and white oaks (Anderson et al, 1993).

American ginseng has a colorful history. It was used by native Americans in their medicine, although for reducing fevers and the like rather than as a general restorative or panacea. For example, the Cherokee used the root for colic, convulsions, dysentery, and headache (Duke, 1989). As for the discovery of American ginseng in North America and its subsequent introduction into China, there have been many accounts (Foster & Chongxi, 1992; Duke, 1989; Bigelow, 1817).

According to some of these stories, a French Jesuit priest living in China, Pére Jartoux, traveled through Manchuria and near what is now Korea in the early 1700s. In 1714 he published his "The Description of the Tartarian Plant Ginseng" in the *Philosophical Transactions of the Royal Society of London*. Father Jartoux seemed to have a favorable impression of the effects of ginseng, using it himself. In his article, he described the fervor with which the Chinese sought the plant in the woods of their home country, described the plant and incidentally said of it that "...if it is to be found in any other country in the world, it may be particularly in Canada, where the forest and mountains, according to the relation of those that have lived there, very much resemble these here." A copy of Jartoux's article reached another Jesuit missionary in Canada, Père Joseph François Lafitau (1681-1746) about 1715. The priest had come to the new world in 1711 to work for six years with the Caughnawage band of Mohawks in Sault Saint Louis, near Montreal. After reading the account of ginseng, he began a systematic search of the woods around the area where he lived, and one day stumbled upon it by accident near his cabin. Lafitau sent samples of the new American ginseng back to China, and soon a vibrant herbal trade ensued beginning in 1718, involving native Americans, frontiersmen like Daniel Boone, French fur traders, and others. To this day, American ginseng, now cultivated, is a major export from the United States and Canada to China, and its cultivation is now increasing dramatically.

The Chinese esteem American ginseng (*Panax quinquefolius*), considering it more "cooling" than Chinese ginseng (*Panax ginseng*) and more of a balanced tonic for Yin as well as Yang. I think American ginseng is especially appropriate for American people because it can help counteract stress, while supporting the adrenal system and strengthening digestion. This can lead to higher energy levels. Ameri-

AMERICAN GINSENG—AN ENDANGERED SPECIES?

The question of whether ginseng provides all the health benefits ascribed to it doesn't seem to be an important factor in the eagerness with which it is harvested from the wilds of the eastern United States. As previously mentioned, American ginseng has been collected commercially and shipped to markets in Asia since the early 1700s, and Daniel Boone talked about collecting it in his memoirs. As herbal medicine has become more popular in North America, wild ginseng has been harvested for domestic markets as well. Today, the vast stands of many native North American medicinal plants have been severely depleted, and none more than ginseng, golden seal, and echinacea, the three herbs that experience the highest demands.

The problem is the price—it keeps going up. Currently, authentic wild American ginseng can sell for as much as $400-600/lb.

In parts of rural Eastern United States and Southern Canada, collecting ginseng, or "sang" as it is popularly called, is still a way of life for some. The location of choice patches are passed on from generation to generation, and their care is considered a matter of great responsibility. Roots should be harvested only when the bright red fruits are ripe and can be replanted to maintain and even expand the wild stands. This is a perfect example of sustainable harvest.

Unfortunately, not all ginseng harvesters are as conscious about the fragility of the natural ecosystem and the wisdom of wild cultivation. High prices and depressed local economies have attracted another sort of picker—those who have no concern for sustainability, but only care to make a quick buck and move on to something else. This kind of harvesting has helped bring ginseng to the brink of extinction in many areas of eastern North America. Field studies by botanical researchers have consistently shown that unprotected wild ginseng sites have lower population counts and set fewer seeds (Anderson et al, 1993). Ginseng is currently threatened or endangered in Kentucky (Sole

cans today with their fast-paced lifestyles are sadly in need of such support. Albert Y. Leung, a natural products researcher in the U.S. who was born in Hong Kong, in his book *Chinese Herbal Remedies* (1984), writes of the differences between Oriental and American ginsengs. He says they are

> *two distinctly different drugs used for different purposes in Chinese medicines...American ginseng is regarded as having cooling or even cold properties as opposed to the warming or invigorating nature of Oriental ginseng...we took American ginseng on numerous occasions in the summer to cool down. And when one of my sisters had scarlet fever and was under the care of a physician who practiced Western medicine my grandmother gave her American ginseng to help cool her fever, with the consent of the doctor. My sister recovered with no complications...if one*

---

et al, 1983), Tennessee (Schmalzer et al, 1985), Virginia (Pae, 1993), and Illinois (Monoson & Schertz, 1985). Virginia state inspectors alone certified more than 14,500 pounds of wild ginseng for export to Asia in 1992, which was 42% over the previous year (Pae, 1993).

Wild American ginseng does not lend itself well to overharvesting. Like many indigenous plants, it is slow-growing and the seeds have a low germination rate (Lewis & Zenger, 1982), but after two years the rate can be as high as 66% (Anderson et al, 1993). Commercial ginseng is ideally harvested after six years of growth, and I have seen many wild roots in commercial trade that were three to seven years old. Because ginseng does not reach reproductive maturity before eight years old (Carpenter & Cottam, 1983), premature harvesting will obviously lead to rapid depletion of wild populations. Ginseng fruit does not mature in many areas before September 1st, so it should not be harvested too early in the year. In many states, permits are required for harvesting, and guidelines are set forth for collectors as to the time of year and age of roots that are allowed to be taken.

If the future sounds bleak for wild American ginseng, there is one bright spot. Many of the wild populations grow in inaccessible places in the southern Appalachians. In fact, hunting wild ginseng can be hazardous to one's health! A long-time picker noted that the wild bears, snakes, and hogs are abundant and are not too pleasant to run into, especially for amateurs who are untrained in the art of survival (Goolick, 1983). He reflects, *"Most people who weren't raised up in it make their first trip and they're cured."*

In some areas of Eastern North America, pollution may also be taking a toll. Ginseng is known to be injured by ozone and sulfur dioxide. These ubiquitous chemicals are spread over large areas by air currents and have contributed to the decline in the health of many ecosystems. Recent computer models have shown that pollution generated from industrial centers in western Pennsylvania, Ohio, and Kentucky can contribute to air, soil, and water contamination as far away as Chesapeake Bay (Nemecek, 1996).

takes ginseng without knowing which type it is, one may use the wrong type and not derive benefits from its effects.

There are several other ginsengs from the genus *Panax* used in Asian medicine. One is *Panax pseudo-ginseng* or *Panax notoginseng* (Burk.) F.H. Chen, which is also called "Tienqi ginseng". It is widely used in Chinese medicine, although it is used not as a tonic primarily, but as a specific to move blood and reduce pain. In Chinese medicine, practitioners consider that any pain in the body is due to "blood stagnation." The blood is not moving properly, so tissues (such as skeletal muscles) do not receive enough nourishment in the form of oxygen, minerals, and sugar, and waste products cannot be removed properly. Tienqi is thought to help correct

American Ginseng, the Cooling Ginseng

The cooling nature of American ginseng also makes it especially useful for North Americans who tend to have too much "heat" in their bodies. By heat it is meant that one's adrenals and thyroid gland are "pushing" the body's metabolism too hard, resulting in chronic inflammation or the accumulation of heat in an organ or organ system. This is often caused by stress arousal from noise, fast-living, overworking, and the use of stimulants like coffee, tea, cola drinks, and products that contain refined sugar. For instance, substances that create liver heat include alcohol, spicy foods, red meat, and various stimulants. Over the months and years of exposure to these, the liver can become overheated, a condition called "liver fire" in TCM. This can in turn lead to such symptoms as chronic headaches, red, dry eyes, irritability for no reason, and eventually hepatitis and cirrhosis.

this. The herb is also famous for controlling bleeding. The two main actions of this herb, though seemingly contradictory, can be explained by looking closely at its proven physiological actions. Animal studies show that Tienqi ginseng may work to stop bleeding through its action on blood coagulation time, while decreasing blood stagnation by dilating blood vessels and reducing capillary permeability. The latter action might help regulate the amount of fluid that seeps out of the capillaries, reducing "stagnation" of blood and water in the tissues.

There are a few more minor *Panax* ginsengs in common use. *Panax japonicum*, or Japanese ginseng, is used to strengthen the stomach, disperse phlegm, and as a tonic. *Panax majoris* Burkhill Ting, known as Pearl ginseng, is also used for deficient Qi, as well as for dispelling lung heat, in conditions such as asthma or cough, though it is not considered as strong or effective as *Panax ginseng* (Hsu et al, 1986).

As previously mentioned, there are several herbs that are unrelated botanically to the *Panax* ginsengs, yet are used for similar purposes. Codonopsis (*Codonopsis pilosula*), called "dang shen," is a good example of this. Like ginseng, it contains saponins, although not ginsenosides, and it is used to increase overall body resistance, boost energy, and improve digestion (Hsu et al, 1986), but it is also famous for increasing the vitality of the lungs. It is much cheaper than ginseng and is more commonly used in soups and stews on a regular basis. It is a widely used mild Qi tonic, good for digestion and less stimulating than ginseng. Many Chinese patent (pre-made commercial) formulas substitute codonopsis for ginseng because it can be taken by young and old alike and is less likely to overstimulate when used to excess. It is also less expensive, which is a great advantage when considering good red Korean ginseng can sell for $20-40/lb or much more, depending on the quality grade, whereas codonopsis is $5-15/lb.

Another herb important to mention is Glehnia, which is in the parsley family and is a good yin (vital essence) tonic as well as a good Qi (vital energy) tonic. It is a common ingredient in Chinese herb prescriptions, especially where there is excess heat in the body, leading to such symptoms and syndromes as rashes, arthritis, acne, or headaches. Glehnia works as a gentle tonic to strengthen the vitality of the body and support the adrenal system.

Prince's ginseng is another useful "ginseng". Its botanical name is *Pseudostellaria heterophylla* Pax ex Pax et Hoffm. and is again not in the ginseng family but in the carnation family, Caryophyllaceae. It is not as stimulating as herbs from the genus *Panax*, especially red ginseng. We will have more on the uses, folklore, and science behind these functionally, but not botanically, related "ginsengs" later in this book.

Finally, last but certainly not least, there is *Eleutherococcus senticosus*, or eleuthero, also called "Siberian ginseng" in the herb industry. This is not a member of the specific genus of the ginsengs, *Panax*, although it is a member of the larger ginseng family, *Araliaceae*. It also contains saponins and other unrelated compounds, dubbed "eleutherosides," rather than "ginsenosides."

In the 1950s a scientist by the name of I.I. Brekhman, a Russian medical doctor, was looking for a source of *Panax ginseng*. Having the Russian love of ginseng but wishing to avoid its expense, Brekhman started looking for other sources and began testing eleuthero, a common plant of the Eastern Russian forests. Eleuthero is a very large plant compared to the rather diminutive ginseng and is faster-growing, both big advantages. After 20 years or so of intensive research he found that it has amazing adaptogenic properties, meaning it helps the body normalize all its functions and adapt to stress. Eleuthero is good for people who are stressed-out or run-down, people who engage in strenuous sports or are on a training program, or are undergoing changes in their lives. Eleuthero is not used for weak digestion like ginseng is; it is used for counteracting stress and regulating different body functions, like blood sugar, or for increasing the oxygenation of the cells and tissue of the body.

With so many true ginsengs having different therapeutic properties based on how they are processed, and other botanically unrelated "ginsengs" that are used for similar purposes, it is not surprising that many people are confused about whether they would benefit from ginseng, and, if so, what kind. To help clarify the different energies and uses, let's look more closely at the nature of the ginsengs—their chemistry and pharmacology. First, we'll consider the Panaxes, Oriental and American, and then Eleuthero. Later, we'll have some information on the other "ginsengs."

THE NATURE OF THE TRUE GINSENGS

If there is a "true" ginseng, it can be defined as a medicinal plant from the ginseng family (Araliaceae) and the genus *Panax*. As we will see, there are only a few plants that meet this criteria, most notably, *Panax ginseng* from the Orient and *Panax quinquefolius* from North America. Taking this definition one step further, the "true" true ginseng can be said to be *P. ginseng*, the illustrious ancient remedy of legend and lore for thousands of years. Though it is probably true that American ginseng, *P. quinquefolius*, possesses some of the same constituents and properties, it does not have the extremely long history of use behind it. We will look at these ginsengs in following sections.

For a more in-depth look at the chemistry and pharmacology (how ginseng acts in the body), practitioners, researchers, writers, or other interested readers are referred to Appendix D (Chemical Constituents of Ginseng and The Pharmacology of Ginseng).

Support for Health Claims–Reviewing Human Studies

In the following sections, we summarize the human clinical studies and reports that are available on ginseng. The results must be reviewed with the knowledge that the methodologies and procedures of the studies vary widely. Some appear to be well-designed and up to modern scientific standards. Others are simply clinical reports and are not placebo-controlled or blinded in any way. Blinding involves preventing the researchers or volunteers from knowing which group is receiving the ginseng and which the placebo. Some of the studies include a very small number of patients, and others larger numbers.

ANTI-STRESS EFFECT

By "toning" the hormonal system, ginseng may help the body retain balance under conditions of stress. It helps the body adapt to stress. Another word for that kind of substance is an "adaptogen." As Dr. Shibata has written,

> In comparison with the effects of usual stimulants, the antifatigue action of ginseng shows an essential difference. The stimulants give effects under most situations, whereas ginseng reveals its action only under the challenge of stress (Shibata et al, 1985).

As detailed under the section "Who Shouldn't Take Ginseng," it is best to avoid ginseng during episodes of acute stress. Ginseng and other adaptogens work best after long-term (one-three months) moderate use by regulating hormone levels and other biological functions to protect us against the damaging effects of chronic stress.

PERFORMANCE-ENHANCEMENT

Despite the difficulties in measuring the effects of an adaptogenic herbal remedy and its subtle to moderately active, multi-system effects, ginseng appears to improve performance, both physical and mental, under conditions of stress, which the following human studies explore (Chong and Oberholzer, 1988).

Physical Performance

➤ A group of researchers from the Institute for the Prophylaxis of Circulatory Diseases at the University of Munich (Germany), conducted by Drs. Imre Forgo, Gustav Schimert, and others, spent more than three years studying the effect of a standardized ginseng extract (G115, standardized to 4% ginsenosides) on the performance of athletes (Forgo & Schemata, 1985), with favorable results (Forgo et al, 1981).

➤ In a 1982 study, the same researchers found that a group of fourteen healthy male athletes who trained at least ten hours/week with a trainer and were receiving the ginseng extract 2 x daily showed an increase in their maximum oxygen uptake, when compared with an equally well-trained placebo group. The ginseng group also had a faster recovery period and lower serum lactate values, which is a measure of muscle fatigue (p < 0.001).

➤ Similar results were achieved during two earlier studies, both of 9 weeks, with 20 (Forgo et al, 1981) and 30 (Forgo, 1983) young volunteers. In the same study, researchers observed an increase in respiratory forced vital capacity, forced expiatory, and maximum breathing capacity (p < 0.001) in the athletes, which was significantly increased over the placebo group (p < 0.001). This improvement was cited as a possible reason for the overall performance gains. In an interesting follow-up to the study, the researchers determined that the athletes achieved performance and metabolic gains that lasted for three weeks after the ginseng administration was stopped.

➤ A double-blind study of 120 subjects, both male and female, aged 30 to 60 revealed the age-specific benefits of ginseng. In the older subjects, those from 40-60, ginseng (2 capsules/day of G115 extract for 12 weeks) increased the capacity to perform visual and acoustic reaction tests; it also improved pulmonary function, which is interesting, as the traditional Chinese interpretation of ginseng is that it "enters the lung meridian." The improvements were statistically significant compared with the placebo group (p 0.01 - p 0.001). However, in the younger subjects, aged 30 to 40, ginseng had no such effects (Forgo, 1980, Forgo et al, 1981).

➤ A double-blind, randomized, crossover study with 50 healthy male sports teachers between the ages of 21 and 47 years old was conducted. Twenty-five volunteers were given a ginseng preparation twice daily, and another 25 were given a placebo for 6 weeks; the groups were then switched for 6 weeks. The work load and total oxygen consumption were significantly less in the ginseng-preparation group. Even more interesting, at the same work load (for both groups), oxygen consumption, carbon dioxide production, and blood lactate levels were lower in the ginseng-preparation group, suggesting that the volunteers in this group utilized energy more efficiently and had greater endurance (Pieralisi et al, 1991).

➤ In a study of 100 young soldiers in Eastern Siberia, those given

Panax ginseng ran a three kilometer race (a little under two miles) on average 53 seconds faster than those given a similar-tasting placebo.

Mental Performance and Mood Enhancement

➤ Forty-five patients with cerebrovascular deficits (lack of blood flow to the brain) were given the pharmaceutical drug Hydergin (a commonly-prescribed drug for the treatment of cerebrovascular problems), a standardized ginseng extract (G115), or a placebo (Quiroga, 1982). It was found that the ginseng extract improved blood flow by a quotient of 34%, compared with 58% for Hydergin and 0.7% for the placebo group. The blood flow was measured by rheography.

➤ Two hundred patients suffering from moderate to severe cerebrovascular insufficiency related to arteriosclerosis were given two 500 mg capsules of a standardized ginseng extract (G115) (Quiroga & Imbriano, 1979). Only 20 patients received a placebo capsule. The patients included 155 men and 45 women from the ages of 41-70, with an average age of 57. Thorough physical exams, including rheoencephalograms, were used to arrive at the diagnoses. The results showed that 36% of the patients had "very favorable" improvement in carotid and cerebral blood flow, 54% had small improvements in the elasticity of the arteries and in blood flow, and 10% had no response. The researchers speculated that ginseng may be well-suited as a daily supplement in the elderly, perhaps combined with other "vasoprotective" substances. *Ginkgo biloba* L. extract is an herb that has extensive research to its credit for this use.

➤ Thirty-eight dental students received up to 14 doses within 30 days of either a placebo, red ginseng root, or American ginseng in a double-blind test. Mathematical performance was not altered in any of the groups, nor were the concentrations of steroids (norepinephrine, cortisol, etc.). Proofreading error detection, mood enhancement, and an anti-fatigue effect were noticed, but the difference from placebo was not particularly significant (Johnson et al, 1980).

➤ Thirty-two wireless operators and telegraphists (age 21-23) were tested for mental concentration and coordination in a double-blind study (Bae, 1978). Those taking ginseng made fewer mistakes (31% down to 17%).

➤ In one double-blind study, in which neither the subjects nor the experimenters knew who was taking ginseng, 30 students were asked to trace, on paper, a complex spiral maze and to select certain letters from randomized groups of letters according to special rules. Those who took ginseng performed better, but the difference was not statistically significant (Sandberg, 1974).

➤ A dozen British nurses, both male and female, whose mood and psychophysiological performance were affected by night duty in a London hospital were studied. They were given either Korean white ginseng or a similar white-powder placebo for three days. The nurses who took ginseng were both more alert and more tranquil during their work and performed better during a test of speed and coordination. Though the results were not statistically significant, the ginseng did have a consistently higher antifatigue effect over placebo and was able to normalize blood sugar raised by stress (Hallstrom et al, 1982).

➤ In a double-blind study with 60 volunteers aged 22-80 years old, Dörling (1980) found that commercial ginseng preparations improved reaction time, two-hand coordination, and physical fitness.

➤ Another controlled study was performed with 120 postoperative gynecological patients. The purified ginsenoside Rg-1 (230 mg) was given daily to the patients, and 60 patients were given a placebo. Serum hemoglobin and total protein, as well as the hematocrit and body weights, were significantly increased in the group receiving ginseng over the control group (Shibata et al, 1985).

➤ In a double-blind, placebo-controlled clinical study, a special ginseng extract preparation (G115, 100 mg 2 X daily for 12 weeks) enhanced attention, mental processing, integrated sensory-motor function, and auditory reaction time in the ginseng group, which consisted of 32 male volunteers aged 20-24 years old. The enhancement in mental processing (mental arithmetic) between the ginseng and placebo groups was statistically-significant (D'Angelo et al, 1986).

➤ Elderly patients were given a standardized ginseng extract (G115) to determine the overall effect on vitality, rigidity, alertness, concentration, visual/motor coordination, grasp of abstract concepts, and positive outlook (Revers et al, 1976). In the double-blind test, either the ginseng extract or a placebo was given to the patients for 90 days. A significant difference in the ginseng group in the above parameters was noted.

➤ In a group of 540 volunteers, significant improvements were seen compared to placebo in subjective and objective parameters, evaluated by an extensive group of tests (Schmidt et al, 1978). Noteworthy was a normalization of blood pressure in volunteers with hypertension, and also of blood sugar levels.

CHRONIC FATIGUE SYNDROME

Besides being useful in helping to increase mental and physical performance, ginseng shows promise for sufferers of chronic fatigue syndrome, helping to counteract the devastating effects of stress and overwork on the nervous and hormonal systems. Chronic fatigue, or asthenia, is a condition brought on by stress, overwork, and disease characterized by a chronic lack of energy and a decline in mental and physical ability. Chronic fatigue is occurring in epidemic proportions in many industrial nations. In one prospective cohort study, 19% of the 4,000 members of a Seattle-based health maintenance organization reported symptoms of chronic fatigue syndrome (Buchwald et al, 1995). These results point to the possibility that millions of people have to deal with chronic fatigue at least some time in their adult life.

In keeping with the present subject, we might understandably ask the question, "Can regular use of ginseng reduce chronic fatigue and help reverse other symptoms commonly associated with the syndrome?" In one group of patients, researchers identified the following symptoms: reduced mental alertness, emotional lability, lack of motivation and initiative, irritability, hostility, indifference to surroundings, unsociability, uncooperative behavior, lack of personal care and hygiene, and lack of appetite (Rosenfeld et al, 1989). These patients were given a placebo and then a standardized ginseng extract (G115) for 56 days. Through a number of psychometric tests designed to evaluate psychological and physical status, it was determined that the patients were improved in many of the areas studied, especially levels of attention and concentration. The change was statistically significant ($p < 0.01$).

SEXUAL ENHANCEMENT AND HORMONAL EFFECTS

Ginseng may also have an effect on sex hormones, which could help explain its traditional use to support sexual energy in older people, but this is far from settled. Traditional Chinese medical texts claim that ginseng... "'enriches the juices and blood of the body' and 'strengthens exhausted sperm and impotent genitals'" (Huang, 1993). So far, scientific evidence to support this particular traditional use for a sexual hormone effect from ginseng is scanty. Experiments do show that ginseng can affect the sexual function and speed sexual maturity of mice and rabbits, not directly by acting as sexual hormones themselves, but by stimulating the hypothalamus-pituitary axis, which in turn signals increased secretion of gonadotropins and sex hormones (Huang, 1993; Chang & But, 1986). One animal test showed that ginseng saponins can increase blood levels of prolactin (a hormone that stimulates the production of progesterone in the ovaries) significantly (Huang, 1993). Another found that blood testosterone levels in rats were significantly increased, and their prostate size was reduced after 30 days with an addition of 5% ginseng to the diet (Fahim et al, 1982). Researchers also found that a ginseng extract could reduce abnormally-high levels of estradiol (the most potent estrogen-like hormone) in the blood of rats (Bespalov et al, 1993). A number of other studies from Russia and China on this aspect of ginseng's activity have been published (Huang, 1993).

When considering how these animal studies correlate with sexual hormone activity in humans, it is important to note how the ginseng was given to the animals, and at what dose. In some of the above studies, the ginseng extracts were administered by injection. Büchi & Jenny (1984) have commented that the blood levels of active ginsenosides achieved by injection in these studies cannot be reached by the oral route based on the low (20%) absorption of the ginsenosides from the gut and other factors. They determined that the maximum blood levels of ginsenosides that could be achieved is less than 1M (a very low level). The study quoted above (Fahim et al, 1982) that demonstrated an increased blood testosterone level in rats after giving them a diet consisting of 5% ginseng powder is suggestive. But considering a moderate food intake for humans of 16 ounces of food/day, one would have to consume about 27 grams of ginseng powder to match the amount given in the study. Even if a more potent extract was used for consumption, it would be difficult to achieve this level of ginsenoside intake. Though what the effect of chronic ginseng use is on blood levels of ginsenosides, the production of testosterone- or estrogen-like compounds, or the stimulation of sexual hormone receptor sites is currently unknown.

Although one Korean author reports that ginseng contains estradiol, estriol, and estrone (Kim 1978), again, it is more likely that the estrogenic effect (if any) is through indirectly stimulating the body's production of estrogen. If estrogen-like compounds are present in ginseng, they occur in minute quantities that are unlikely to be active in humans. There are numerous published analyses of ginseng that make no mention of any of these compounds. Like other adaptogens, ginseng may have the ability to regulate and balance the levels of estrogen in the body by indirect regulatory action.

There are few human trials that study the effect of ginseng on hormonal function. One placebo-controlled study of 144 women showed that "ginseng completely eliminated distressing menopausal symptoms in 60% of the patients, compared with 19% in the placebo group" (Owen, 1981). It is unknown whether the outcome was related to an estrogen-modulating effect, but the study does suggest a hormonal-regulating effect of some kind. In another study researchers failed to detect any changes in luteinizing hormone (LH), follicle-stimulating hormone (FSH), estrogen or testosterone in 60 male and 60 female volunteers ages 30-60 after giving them 2 capsules/day of a standardized ginseng extract (Forgo et al, 1981). Likewise, hormonal effects were not noted in a study by the same group with 30 top class

THE STRANGE CASE OF GINSENG FACE CREAM

A 44-year-old patient got more than she bargained for after using a ginseng face cream from China (Hopkins et al, 1988). She had passed through menopause two years earlier and noticed the symptoms of vaginal dryness, hot flashes, and a cessation of bleeding. Her follicle-stimulating hormone (FSH) level was 105 mIU/ml of serum. After using the Fang Fang ginseng face cream during the winter months, she experienced 2 episodes of spotting and had her FSH levels checked again—they had dropped to 36 mIU/ml (normal levels for menstruating women is 4-30 mIU/ml). She discontinued the face cream and one month later the bleeding had stopped and her FSH levels had returned to 70 mIU. Three weeks after beginning the face cream again her FSH had dropped again to 27 mIU, and 1 week later she had another episode of uterine bleeding. Since then, the patient has not used the face cream. Her FSH levels have risen and she has not had further bleeding periods.

Does this case add credence to the case for ginseng as an estrogen stimulant? Were the ginsenosides absorbed through the skin regulating the woman's hormonal levels? It is an interesting question and one that cannot be answered definitively, because the face cream was apparently not analyzed for synthetic steroids. Chinese patent formulas are known to contain synthetic drugs upon occasion, and even products manufactured in North America can contain a small amount of synthetic progesterone (below 0.5%) without being labeled as such. If the seeming hormonal activity was caused by ginseng active constituents, it brings up some interesting possibilities.

male athletes, age 18 to 31 years old after 9 weeks (Forgo, 1983).

Based on a knowledge of the way adaptogens work, if production of sex hormones is adequate in an individual, stimulating the homeostatic hormone control center (the hypothalamus-pituitary-adrenal axis) isn't likely to increase production of sex hormones. Its use in the old, but not the young—the traditional use—would seem to make the most sense.

Though science has not conclusively shown ginseng to have a sexual hormone-like action in humans, the traditional use of ginseng in this regard continues to engage interested researchers to demonstrate this effect. As we age, the ability of our bodies to make the hormones and other substances that keep us functioning normally tends to decline. *Panax ginseng* has always had a reputation for being useful for older people, in order to help stoke the hormonal fires of life. That is how it is used in China. Indeed, one common saying in China is worth remembering: "If you use ginseng when you are young, what will you use when you are old?"

LONGEVITY BENEFITS

Ginseng has a long-standing reputation as an anti-aging and anti-senility remedy. This is perhaps true, based on its proven ability (at least in animals) to increase the production of various hormones, enhance nerve regeneration, and a number of other effects discussed above. Ginseng extracts may also be able to facilitate the uptake and utilization of life-giving oxygen to the tissues and organs. In one study, European researchers studied the oxygen status with 63 volunteers (Von Ardenne et al, 1987) by using a variety of measurements. It was found

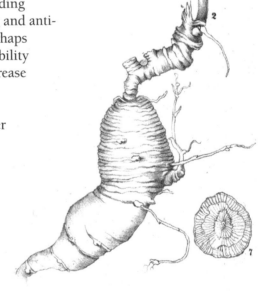

Panax quinquefolius – root and 'neck' showing tight ridges of a wild root from *American Medicinal Plants* by C. Millspaugh, 1887

that a daily dose of 2 capsules of a commercially-available standardized extract (G115) for 4 weeks could increase the resting pO_2 uptake by the body as well as oxygen transport into the organs and tissues by about 29%.

However, can ginseng prolong life in healthy animals or humans by extending the life span of the body's cells and allowing them to continue reproduction and maintain vigor beyond their genetic programming? So far, the scientific evidence for humans is not compelling. Ginseng *does* seem to have the ability to help prevent some diseases, and thus prolong life in this sense. Animal studies have not supported the longevity factor in healthy older animals, but can prolong the life of young female mice (Huang, 1993). Only a few studies on the anti-senility effects of ginseng have been performed on humans, all in China.

In one study, a group of 358 patients 50-85 years old received a sugar-coated tablet of purified ginsenosides (50 mg) 3 x daily orally for two months (Zhao, 1990). Another group of 123 patients received a sugar-coated placebo (starch) pill. The researchers reported that patients in the ginseng group experienced significant improvement of memory and an increase in white blood cells and other immune functions. The ginsenosides appeared to help relieve symptoms of angina pectoris and heart irregularities (pre-ventricular and pre-auricular contractions) better than the placebo pill.

IMMUNE-STRENGTHENING EFFECTS

The effects of ginseng extracts on the human immune system were tested by European researchers in a double-blind study with 3 groups of 20 volunteers (Scaglione et al, 1990). Group A took a capsule containing 100 mg of an aqueous extract of ginseng every 12 hours for 8 weeks, group B a capsule of lactose, and group C a capsule with 100 mg of a standardized ginseng extract (G115). Blood samples were taken at the beginning of the trial, at 4 weeks, and at 8 weeks. Chemotaxis of PMNs, the phagocytosis index (PHI), and phagocytosis fraction (PHF) were enhanced at 4 weeks, but more significantly at 8 weeks. The standardized extract group had a significantly stronger response, and the placebo group showed a less marked response only in PHI and PHF at 8 weeks. Total lymphocytes (T3), T helper (T4) subset, suppresser cells (T8) subset counts, and the T4/T8 ratio showed a significant enhancement only in the ginseng group B over placebo ($p<0.05$). Moreover, blastogenesis of circulating lymphocytes and natural killer-cell activity (NK) were significantly enhanced, according to the researchers.

RELIEF OF HANGOVER SYMPTOMS AND
INCREASED ALCOHOL CLEARANCE

Ginseng has demonstrated the ability to enhance the breakdown and elimination of ethyl alcohol in animals (Lee et al, 1993). Researchers studied this effect in a group of 14 healthy human volunteers. Each participant was used as his/her own control, that is they were tested separately with and without ginseng 40 minutes after receiving the same amount of alcohol. The blood alcohol was, on average, 35% lower when the volunteers were given the ginseng extract.

USE IN MEDICINE: HEART DISEASE AND CANCER

As one might imagine, ginseng is commonly used throughout China in hospitals to treat a variety of diseases, especially cancer, heart disease, and diabetes. If we want to review what science has to say about the efficacy of this use, we must look into clinical studies from China since there are few, if any, controlled clinical trials performed in the west.

Heart Disease

In one uncontrolled human study (Ding et al, 1995), red ginseng was given to patients with class IV congestive heart failure. A total of 45 patients were divided into 3 equal groups. The first group was given red ginseng only, the second, dioxin (a cardiac stimulant from the foxglove or digitalis plant), and the third group a combination of the two. Groups 2 and 3 showed the best improvement in hemodynamical and biochemical indexes. No side effects of the red ginseng treatment were noted. The researchers concluded that red ginseng was an effective adjuvant for the treatment of congestive heart failure.

Researchers in China have also given total ginsenosides to patients after open heart surgery, compared to a similar group not using the compounds (Zhan, 1994). They report better recovery and less tissue damage due to ischemia (lack of oxygen) in the patients who received the ginsenosides.

Regular ginseng use might help cut cholesterol and triglyceride levels according to animal studies and one human clinical report. Japanese researchers found that oral administration of red ginseng powder reduced plasma total cholesterol, triglyceride, and NEFA, while elevating plasma HDL-cholesterol ("good" cholesterol) (Yamamoto, 1983). Platelet adhesiveness was also reduced by ginseng administration.

A combination product consisting of 60 mg of a 24% standardized

Ginkgo biloba extract and 100 mg of a standardized ginseng extract (4% ginsenosides) was given to 10 patients with a median age of 26 years old. European researchers reported that the systolic and diastolic blood pressure in both groups was significantly reduced (Kiesewetter, 1992). Improved blood flow was seen by observing an increased red blood cell velocity in the nail-fold capillaries.

Cancer

A group of researchers performed statistical analysis on 1987 pairs of human volunteers to determine the preventive effect of ginseng intake against various human cancers (Yun & Choi, 1995). The individuals in one of the groups were diagnosed with various cancers; those in the other were healthy. They determined that ginseng users had a lower risk of cancers of the lip, oral cavity, pharynx, esophagus, stomach, colorectal area, liver, pancreas, larynx, lungs, and ovaries. There was no improvement in the risk factor for cancers of the female breast, uterine cervix, urinary bladder, and thyroid gland. Smokers who used ginseng regularly had a lower risk of cancer. In a follow-up study, the same researchers compared two groups of 905 patients and found a statistically (p less than 0.01) significant lower incidence of cancer in the ginseng users (Yun & Choi, 1990). The researchers apparently did not take into account such factors as diet and other health habits in the study. It is possible that people taking the time to use ginseng also had better habits in other regards. Still, the study is suggestive and merits follow-up studies.

In China, immune adjuvant therapy with herbal medicine is commonly used with chemo and radiation therapy. One of the studies reported the use of ginseng leaf and the root of *Astragalus membranaceous* Bunge Fabaceae (huang qi) in conjunction with such chemotherapeutic agents as vincristine, cyclophosphamide, methotrexate, and carmustine for treating patients with small cell lung cancer (Cha & Chang, 1994). The researchers reported that their combined treatments raised the survival rates of the patients "considerably," 10 of the 12 patients gaining more than 3-17 years of survival. The treatments were given for more than 2 years.

Other Medical Uses

A research group in Europe (Zuin, 1987) found that standardized ginseng extract improved values on liver screening tests in a group of elderly patients with chronic liver disease due to chronic use of drugs and alcohol. The results were superior to those seen in a similar group of patients taking a placebo, but the difference was not statistically significant. Since there are a number of other herbal remedies for liver support (milk thistle (*Silybum marianum* [L.] Gaertn.), ginger (*Zingiber officinale* Roscoe), schisandra (*Schisandra chinensis* [Turcz.]), turmeric (*Curcuma longa* L.), artichoke leaf (*Scolymus*), etc., ginseng may be considered to be of minor importance. However, if useful for other purposes, it can be added to a regimen for liver health.

Ginseng and Pregnancy

Ginseng consumption during pregnancy is a long-established tradition in China and thought to supply extra energy to the mother as well as the baby. In one study of eighty-eight women who took ginseng during their pregnancies, the incidence of preeclampsia (a form of toxemia in pregnancy) was lower in the ginseng group than in the control group (Chin, 1991). Although no adverse effects were reported in those who took ginseng, pregnant women should take note of the following precautions, particularly in the use of red ginseng:

1. Consulting a health practitioner is recommended before taking ginseng during pregnancy.
2. Do not exceed recommended dose (3-9 g.)
3. Contraindicated for hypertension
4. Using ginseng may potentiate the effects of caffeine and other stimulants.

THE CONCEPT OF ADAPTOGENS

In 1988, I had the good fortune to meet with Dr. Israel I. Brekhman, a physician who for many years was director of the Institute of the Physiology and Pharmacology of Adaptation in Vladivostok, Russia. It was his first trip to the United States. The occasion was an international conference on ginseng.

The meeting was held in a place where adaptation might be somewhat of a challenge, especially for a person coming from Vladivostok in the remote far east of Russia. It was in Las Vegas. The meeting was held in a noisy, glittering casino. Rows of flashing and whirring slot machines were being hopefully, and somewhat vacantly, caressed. Dr. Brekhman was wearing a suit, a camera suspended from his neck. He looked somewhat out of place and a little bewildered, yet he also looked very kind and had a presence about him.

I knew him previously only by his international reputation and his many articles on eleuthero and adaptogens. I had also read his unusual and interesting work, *"Man and Biologically Active Substances,"* in which he details how pollution and modern stresses can affect our immune system and general health, and how natural substances, such as ginseng and eleuthero, can help us survive and maintain health.

The work, published in 1980, was well ahead of its time. It emphasized the need to study the science and art of health, not disease. His work over the last 40 years has shown that because most of us hover in a state somewhere between health and disease, we need a group of nature's gifts called adaptogens, which work by helping move us toward health.

Brekhman turned out to be warm, open, energetic, and vigorous, with a good sense of humor. He told me that in Russia, many medical doctors prescribe herbs in their practices—especially in the outlying districts. He began to study eleuthero because the Russian people have strongly accepted the concept that a natural remedy can help bolster innate resistance to disease and help prevent stress from taking such a devastating toll on our nervous, hormonal, and immune systems. *Panax ginseng* is very popular, but it is scarce and mostly too expensive for people to take on a daily basis.

So he began to test other members of the ginseng family in his research center. Since this beginning, in 1959, thousands of tests have been done on eleuthero and other herbal adaptogens. Literally hundreds of thousands of people have taken these natural strengtheners, which have shown remarkable effectiveness for preventing a variety of ailments, increasing stamina and sports performance, and helping us adapt to changing conditions in our environment.

The word "adaptogen" was coined in 1947 by Brekhman's teacher, the Russian scientist, N.V. Lazarev. In his view, an adaptogen has to fulfill three criteria. The substance or therapy must:

1. Be innocuous and cause minimal disorders in the physiological functions of an organism.

2. Show a nonspecific action, that is, increase resistance to adverse influences by a wide range of physical, chemical, and biochemical factors.

3. Exert a normalizing action irrespective of the direction of the pathologic state.

Although Lazarev's original work on adaptogens was carried out with a chemical substance, dibazole, subsequent work by Brekhman focused on ginseng (*Panax ginseng*) and later, eleuthero or Siberian ginseng (*Eleutherococcus senticosus*). Besides herbs, other adaptogens are recognized for their normalizing and general strengthening effects—for instance, saunas and cold water (when properly applied) and all forms of exercise, and as Norman Cousins has so eloquently put forth, laughing. Today, more than ever, we need these kinds of substances.

The adaptogens have been shown to act in certain ways to protect and strengthen people in a variety of life situations against stress. Generally, these include the following:

1. Support adrenal function, counteract weakening effects of stress.
2. Enable the cells of our body to have access to more energy.
3. Help the cells eliminate toxic metabolic by-products.
4. Provide an anabolic effect, used by body-builders.
5. Help the body utilize oxygen more efficiently.
6. Strengthen proper regulation of our biorhythms.

Although we can change our environment virtually at will with air-conditioning and lighting and isolate ourselves from noise and other stimuli with buildings of concrete, we risk losing our ability to adapt to changing conditions in the world. The results of this narrowing ability to adapt, brought about by our own cunning, may be our undoing, for the universe is constantly changing. Too, the more we insulate ourselves from environmental change, the more we isolate ourselves from that which gives us life. René Dubos, the humanistic scientist and a special guiding light for me, wrote,

> This state of adaptedness gives a false sense of security because it does not have a lasting value and does not prepare for the future (Dubos, 1965).

Therefore, it seems that the best course for survival is for us to increase our adaptability to our environment, not the other way around. In other words, instead of leaning on air conditioning to adapt to hot weather, it may be best to strengthen ourselves and cultivate flexibility—both of mind and body, and this is where the adaptogens can be of great importance.

The Russian scientist, G.M. Barenboim said it well:

> For the first time in the history of human civilization the biological potentialities of the human body have failed to meet the requirements imposed on it by the epoch. One witnesses an unusual 'epidemic' of fatigue aggravated by the powerful action of man-made, external chemical and physical environmental factors. Like the drugs that saved

the world from numerous bacterial and viral epidemics that cost millions of lives in the past, the adaptogens are needed to help man withstand the diverse stresses of today (Barenboim 1986).

Eleuthero: The Model Adaptogen

Like the true ginsengs, Eleuthero appears to act primarily as an adaptogen (Farnsworth et al, 1985). If the blood sugar is too high, it brings it down; if it is too low, it brings it up. It helps us adapt to higher elevations and changes in time zones (jet lag); it is very good for normalizing the body and protecting it against stress. It also supports the immune system and the adrenal glands. It is milder and not as stimulating as the regular ginsengs, so it can be taken for a longer period of time by people of different ages and constitutional types.

Eleuthero is the best-studied of the adaptogens. With over 35 years of intense clinical and practical research behind it, eleuthero is taken by millions of Russians daily. It is used by the Russian Olympic team, especially weight-lifters and runners. The extract was used by cosmonauts to adapt to the radically-different conditions in outer space. Among others, mountain climbers, sailors, and factory workers all use eleuthero regularly to increase adaptability, reduce sick days, and promote increased endurance. I took eleuthero extract once for a nine-month period and for several shorter periods in the last ten years and noticed a decided increase in endurance and performance.

While many of the Russian studies with people working in factories and other industries were not performed double-blind (preferred by the medical profession and government regulators today), they offer interesting insights into how adaptogens work on large populations of everyday working people and what benefits they might offer.

The following studies were performed on thousands of people in a variety of normal daily working situations, and the results were recorded. In most cases there was no difference in effects noted between men and women taking the extract. Here are some of the studies with normal, healthy volunteers:

➤ The number and speed of radiogram receptions for radiotelegraphic operators were increased with eleuthero daily doses of 1 1/2 droppersful (60 drops) of a liquid extract over a one-month period.

➤ Skiers taking a single dose of eleuthero extract (3 droppersful) before a race increased their resistance to harmful effects of cold and increased physical endurance, especially when a skier was not fully trained.

➤ Workers in a publishing house whose job involved physical labor showed enhanced cardiovascular output, ability to work, and improved appetite, without hypertension. However, the extract was not recommended for people with blood pressure over 180/90 mm Hg.

➤ Proofreaders were more effective in their work after taking 1 1/2 droppersful of eleuthero extract daily for 30 days. (Two studies)

➤ Sailors who took eleuthero extract showed improved work capability and normalization of body functions under conditions of elevated temperatures while on long sea voyages.

➤ One thousand factory workers (in a city of the polar region) who took 3 droppersful of eleuthero extract daily showed an overall 50% reduction in general sickness and 40% reduction in the number of lost work days.

➤ Brekhman studied drivers of heavy trucks who took eleuthero extract in tea for 6 years. The total number of sick people from influenza dropped dramatically over these years, from 41.8 per 100 workers to 2.7. The number of days per year lost because of influenza dropped from 286 per 100 workers to 11. (Other studies showing that eleuthero could dramatically reduce the number of sick days due to influenza among thousands of different workers are reported).

➤ Further studies show that eleuthero extract, when taken on a regular basis, can improve visual and hearing acuity, color perception, increase efficiency in people with jobs requiring attention, and improve physical and mental working capacity under unfavorable climatic conditions (too hot, too cold, high altitude).

Here are some of the studies showing benefits with specific diseases:

➤ Forty-five volunteers with heart disease showed enhanced feelings of well-being, fewer chest pains, reduced blood pressure and cholesterol levels, and improved ECG readings after 6 to 8 courses (25 days each) of eleuthero extract (1 to 1 1/2 droppersful 3 times daily before meals).

➤ In a second study on 65 patients with cardiovascular disease, with the same dose as above, improvements were noted by some after the first course (25-35 days).

➤ Several studies involving patients with diabetes showed that eleuthero extract is effective in lowering serum glucose levels in some cases.

➤ People with both hypotension and hypertension showed normalization of blood pressure after courses of eleuthero extract. Several other studies support these findings.

➤ Fifty-eight people with psychological imbalances having symptoms such as extreme exhaustion, irritability, insomnia, decreased work capacity, and a general state of anxiety showed improvement after two droppersful of eleuthero extract a.m. and p.m. for four weeks. The patients felt that sound sleep and an increase in their sense of well-being were the most important benefits.

➤ Five more studies with nearly 160 neurotic patients showed that eleuthero extract (as little as 1 dropperful a day) can be of benefit (as indicated above). Some of the studies lasted for ten years.

Overall, the studies with human volunteers have helped clarify the broad-spectrum of activity for eleuthero extract. To summarize, the major physiological effects that have been demonstrated by Russian scientists include a strong antitoxic effect (against environmental toxins), a protective effect against radiation, a normalizing effect against hypothermia, a blood-sugar regulating effect, a liver-protective effect, an enhancement of the liver's ability to break down and rid the body of drugs, an increase in the body's ability to resist infection, and adrenal supportive activity.

Most important is eleuthero's positive influence on work capacity and endurance (anti-fatigue effect), increasing the ability of the cells throughout the body to utilize phosphorus-containing energy molecules and deal with lactic acid and other by-products of metabolism (the sore muscles from a heavy workout result from lactic acid buildup). This effect is especially important for athletes, both professional and "weekend" sports enthusiasts alike. For infertile men, eleuthero has shown the ability to increase semen output and reproductive capability.

ORIENTAL, AMERICAN, AND SIBERIAN GINSENGS — A SUMMARY

As we have seen, the different types of "ginseng" can have different properties. *Panax ginseng* is appropriate for certain conditions and for yang-deficient, cold, debilitated, and perhaps older people. *Panax quinquefolius*, or American ginseng, is more balanced and can be used by younger, less debilitated, hotter, stressed people. *Eleuthero*, or Siberian "ginseng," is even more neutral; it acts primarily as a balancing and anti-stress agent and is appropriate for people under stress.

By now, you may have an idea whether one of the ginsengs may be appropriate for you. In the next section, we'll discuss the various forms ginseng comes in and how it is prepared and used.

In the last section, we'll summarize some of the information about the three ginsengs discussed above and explore other herbs often classified with ginseng, either botanically or because they act similarly as energy tonics.

PART TWO:
Ginseng, Maximizing Its Potential

After reviewing some of the many benefits of ginseng, you will hopefully feel enthusiastic about adding a ginseng supplement or tea to your daily health regime. Because ginseng is such a popular herb worldwide, the demand for bulk roots to make tea, as an addition to soups and other foods (a traditional way of using it), and of course convenient commercial products is understandably high.

It is safe to say that not all ginseng products are created equal. Because of the rarity of old roots of good quality, the temptation to substitute inferior roots or even roots of other plants in commercial shipments of the herb is very real—even to the point of selling "spent" material (roots that have the active constituents previously removed) for use in commercial tablets and capsules.

Because it is common knowledge that ginseng products can be of very uneven quality, Mark Blumenthal, the founder of the American Botanical Council (ABC), has initiated a major study of more than 250 commercial ginseng products of all kinds available throughout North America. Results from this monumental study will be published in the journal of ABC, *HerbalGram* (Antoniak, 1994). "Mislabeling of ginseng products has been an issue for more than 20 years," Blumenthal says. "And with the proliferation of ginseng products today we don't really know how many contain what it says on the label." The results will likely show what many herbalists already suspect—it is best to be cautious when choosing a ginseng product. This section discusses some important points to consider when making your choice, from the various sources of ginseng root, optimum age of the roots, and different ways to extract it to maximize the activity.

REGULATORY GUIDELINES FOR GINSENG

Many countries of the world publish an official compendium of herbs and synthetic drugs that are approved for use in medicine by the regulatory body charged with determining quality standards, doses, and appropriate use for those substances. These are generally called

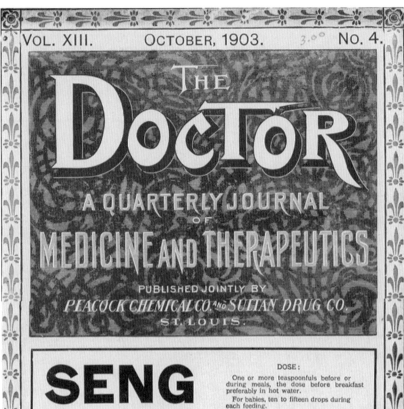
A 1903 ad for a digestant called "Seng"
from "The Doctor, a Quarterly Journal"

Pharmacopeias, and they differ widely in the drugs that are included. Ginseng is still "official" in a number of world pharmacopeias, including those of Austria, China, France, Japan, Russia, and Switzerland (Reynolds, 1993). Several countries call for a minimum amount of ginsenosides (calculated as ginsenoside Rg_1) to be present in ginseng products:

*France: 2%   *Germany: 1.5%   *Switzerland: 1.5%

For a discussion of standard methods used to determine identity, purity, and quality of ginseng, see *The Chinese Pharmacopeia,* English edition (Tu, 1988), or the German pharmacopeia, *DAB 10* (1991).

COMMERCIAL GRADES OF GINSENG, WILD OR CULTIVATED

There are two different schools of thought on commercial ginseng cultivation—commercial chemical-based farming and bio-dynamic organic farming. The roots are also available from the wild in North America, though these resources are rapidly disappearing. Most of the commercial ginseng in the United States is grown around the great lakes and in Canada's British Columbia because of the beneficial climate. For optimum growth and production of active constituents, the plant needs to be warm and moist during the summer and have a good freeze in the winter. If you've ever lived around the Great Lakes, you know that in the summer the humidity gets up around 95%, and the winter temperatures go well below freezing.

Unfortunately, when American or Asian ginseng is grown commercially, the humid conditions make it very susceptible to insect and fungus attack. It is also known that the ginseng plant can severely deplete the soil in which it is growing after several years. Added to the practice of monoculturing ginseng these conditions provide an environment where fungus and insect overgrowth is likely. Farmers using these methods must use heavy doses of synthetic fertilizers, fungicides, pesticides, and herbicides to "protect" their investment. These practices can weaken the immune system of the plants and degrade the quality of the soil, resulting in the continuing dependence on chemical farming (Wolfe, 1995; Fryer, 1995). Commercially-cultivated roots often contain residues of these chemicals that persist in the roots. For instance, a group of Korean researchers found organochlorine pesticide residues in samples of commercially-cultivated ginseng roots. They detected hexachlorobenzene, heptachlor epoxide, and p,p'-DDE, as well as 0.3-1.2 mg/kg of the fungicide quintozene (Kwon et al, 1986). Exposure to fumigants has been shown to affect levels of minerals in harvested ginseng roots (Ahn et al, 1981). Besides its possible harmful effects on the nutrient quality of ginseng and on the people using ginseng (especially with consistent, long-term use), there is some evidence that these chemicals reduce the ginsenoside content, and thus the overall quality of the roots (Wolfe, 1995).

The chemicals, already pervasive in our environment, place a heavy burden on the health of human beings, wild animals, and whole ecosystems. For these reasons, forward-thinking ginseng growers from Wisconsin are concerned about the quality of the roots they are growing and selling and the health of their soil, and they are doing something about it. The organization they have formed is called the Wisconsin Ginseng Crop Improvement Project (WGCIP). Its stated goal is learning to grow ginseng bio-dynamically and organically. They are in the process of developing methods to do this, including the use of seaweeds and other natural fertilizers, and crop rotation. Lee Fryer, one of the pioneers of Wisconsin ginseng cultivation, is enthusiastic about the ability of farmers to respond to the new challenge of environmentally-sound, sustainable agriculture. A great motivational factor is the prospect of improving the quality of the ginseng they grow, with the hope of achieving ginsenoside contents from 8-10% in the harvested root (Fryer, 1995). In the end, we all benefit from this inspirational approach.

Wild ginseng is the most desirable kind of ginseng to many ginseng "heads," but since it is so expensive and rare, the best alternative is what we call "woods-grown ginseng." In this method of cultivation, one-two year old ginseng starts or the ginseng crowns (top of the root) are used. If you want to grow your own ginseng, put one-year old and two- year old roots into well-drained high humus soil in a shady spot next to your house; or if you want to put a bed in, you need to protect it with 30 or 40% shade cloth and keep the roots well-watered. They will grow, but they do like a rich soil and not too much direct exposure to the hot, dry sun. See the Resource Section for where to get information about ginseng cultivation and for sources of ginseng seeds, starts, or crowns.

Woods-grown ginseng is produced by taking the seeds or the small ginseng plants and putting them out in their natural habitat—right in the woods where they would normally grow. Ideally, the young plants are not watered or fertilized, but just watched over as they continue to develop in their natural habitat. They are probably more crowded than they would be in the wild, but good-quality woods-grown ginseng is not cultivated with any commercial fertilizers or pesticides or herbicides.

You can buy woods-grown ginseng for about $65-$100 per pound. For personal use, not that much is needed, so two small roots might be around $10; if they were wild roots, however, the cost would be approximately $50 or $60.

As mentioned above, the top of the root is called the crown, and then there is the body of the root, and then the tail. The tail consists of the long rootlets. Tails are generally much cheaper than other parts of the root. (The very top part of the root where the above-ground plant buds out from is called the neck, "ren shen lu"; it is traditionally used as a mild emetic—an agent to induce vomiting—although in southern and central China it is also considered a tonic, like ginseng root) (Bensky and Gamble, 1986).

THE AGE OF GINSENG

To determine the age of the root, count the scars; each scar represents one year of growth. This method provides an accurate method of determining the age of most ginseng roots (Anderson et al, 1993). Inferior roots don't have the neck attached, so with these you can't tell. A good harvester will want to show you the age of the roots and wouldn't even harvest roots under three years old, as they are not considered worthwhile. For optimum strength, they should be at least three years old and preferably at least six to twelve years old. Between the fourth and sixth years, the root doubles in weight, and the increase in ginsenosides also peaks then, usually by the end of the summer of the fifth year or during the sixth year (Samukawa et al, 1995). After that, the root continues to grow and accumulate the ginsenosides, but more slowly.

Good roots are between six and twelve years old. That's what you would find in commercial trade. The very best roots are fifty to one-hundred years old. When you see one of these old roots, you can see where the name "ren shen," meaning "man root," came from—it looks like a person with a head, a torso, arms, and legs, and in well-preserved roots, the many small rootlets look like lines of energy emanating from the fingers and toes!

MAKING GINSENG REMEDIES AT HOME

Studies show that the alcoholic (ethanolic) extract is about as effective as water in extracting the ginsenosides from ginseng. However, a group of researchers from Korea were able to show that an alcoholic extract had the most active antioxidant properties of any kind of extract (Choi et al, 1983). So whether you prefer to make a tea or a tincture or purchase an extract of ginseng is a matter of personal choice and convenience. The most important factor is the identity, quality, and freshness of the original ginseng that went into the product.

HOW TO DECOCT GINSENG TEA

You are going to get a slightly different constituent profile if you make a tea with hot boiling water than if you make a cold extraction with alcohol and water. Some constituents will be more alcohol soluble; others more water soluble. But if the question is are you going to get a different result by taking a tincture than by taking a tea every day, there isn't enough difference to really worry about, except the tincture is more stimulating and the tea more supportive or nourishing over the long-term (tonifying).

A tea is often used as a tonic and can be used longer term, because a lot of the sugars and polysaccharides (giant sugar molecules which are immune-tonifying), as well as minerals, will come out in the hot water decoction as the cell walls break down. So, in general, teas can be used for a longer period of time, and they are more deeply tonifying; whereas the alcoholic liquid extracts are for a shorter time—maybe a month or two. If you are taking tea, drinking it between mealtimes will give you the most benefit, because it is quickly absorbed and the body doesn't have food constituents to break down and assimilate at the same time.

Some ginseng roots are very hard, and it takes a lot of boiling to get all the essence out—especially for the red ginsengs, which are harder than the white ginsengs. For this reason, dried, sliced red ginseng is available from most Chinese herb dealers. The slices make for an efficient extraction because of the increased surface area. Decocting an herb is a little different from making tea; you bring the herb in water to a boil and then simmer it until only half the water remains. You can double extract it, too; in other words, boil it for 45 minutes in water, pour the tea off, add fresh water, and then boil it for another 1/2 hour. The roots are generally expensive enough that it is desirable to extract all the active ingredients out of the ginseng and not leave any behind.

Traditionally, ginseng is never cooked in a metal pot. This makes sense, because ginseng contains antioxidants, and boiling it in an iron pot might cause iron, an "oxidant," to destroy some of those antioxidants. Use an enamel or glass pot instead. Or you may want to purchase a "ginseng cooker," which is a kind of porcelain or clay double-boiler. If you do buy one, you can use it to artfully decoct any herb.

A tea kept refrigerated will be good for about 4 days. Divide up the tea into several daily doses—morning and evening or morning, afternoon, and evening, if you need a stronger dose. An average dose would be 1 cup, morning and evening.

If you want, you can add some ginger to your ginseng tea. The ginger will make it a little warmer, increase circulation, and strengthen digestion. Try white ginseng with a little ginger, either fresh or dried. Make a decoction of it and have a couple of cups per day. This is a standard remedy for weak, cold digestion.

HOW TO MAKE A TINCTURE OF GINSENG

If taking ginseng in liquid extract form appeals to you, you can make your own tincture. In making liquid extracts, alcohol and water are used to extract the active ingredients from the plant.

Liquid extracts are more convenient than making tea and have excellent keeping qualities. The alcohol will also preserve it for up to three years, so you don't have to worry about fermentation or bacteria or fungi growing in there. Alcohol also preserves the active constituents, because it destroys enzymes that break them down. In plants there are always enzymes, and when a plant is dried, those enzymes become inactive, but as soon as the plant is rehydrated, the enzymes are reactivated and start breaking down the active constituents. Alcohol, however, destroys those enzymes.

Another advantage of a tincture over a tea is that the alcohol will carry the active constituents into the blood system faster, so they are quickly and completely absorbed.

To make your own tincture at home, buy some of the woods-grown roots and grind them up to a smoothie-like consistency in a blender with 80 or 100 proof (40-50% ethanol) vodka. When the solids settle out, make sure there is an inch and a half or two inches of clear vodka over the herb to keep the macerating (soaking) herb from coming in contact with the air, which can lead to fermentation. Make sure to shake the macerating herb blend every day. After two weeks, strain

---

TABLE 2: GUIDELINES FOR GINSENG PRODUCTS

➤ If made properly, tinctures can be an excellent way to take ginseng

➤ Ask the supplement consultant in the herb department or herb store for recommendations regarding quality-conscious companies, as the quality can vary considerably

➤ Powdered extracts in capsules or tablets that are "standardized" to ginsenoside content (at least 5%) can be effective.

➤ Make sure to determine which kind of ginseng(s) are in the product—select the ones that are best-suited for your personal needs.

➤ Make sure to take a ginseng product for at least one month, up to six-nine months for maximum effect. When using ginseng for more than a month, take three-day breaks every few weeks.

➤ When purchasing whole ginseng roots for tea or home preparations, the best quality roots are ones that still have the "neck" (the stalk above the crown that still has the scars from the growth of previous years). Try to select roots that are about four-six years old, which is the optimum age for most purposes. Very old roots can have a higher ginsenoside content, but are often higher priced (Jang et al, 1983).

➤ Instant tea powders and cubes probably are low in ginsenosides. One group of researchers analyzed six commercial samples and found they contained an average of about 1% ginsenosides. Domestic whole tinctures, standardized extracts, and whole good-quality roots are probably a better buy.

and squeeze the herb through a cheesecloth or a linen cloth, and discard (or compost) the spent herb (called the marc). If desired, filter the tincture through an unbleached coffee filter to clarify the liquid. This is only necessary when the tincture is to be placed into dropper bottles, because the small amount of unfiltered solids in your tincture can plug up the fine dropper tip, which I have found to be a nuisance. If you plan to take the extract by the teaspoonful (or one-half teaspoonful 2-3 x daily—a good average dose), then it is preferable to leave the liquid unfiltered, since useful constituents may be filtered out and possibly lost in the process.

Home-made or ready-made commercial ginseng "liqueurs" are a time-honored way to take ginseng, and it even makes scientific sense, as ginsenosides are very soluble in a mixture of 40% water and 60% alcohol (80 proof vodka). (If you avoid alcohol in all forms—if you are a recovering alcoholic, for example, and don't like to keep alcohol in the house—this isn't the best form of ginseng for you. Instead, make a tea or purchase a powdered extract in capsule or tablet form).

To take this alcohol-based tincture of ginseng, take one-half teaspoonful in a little warm water or tea 2-3 x daily. Try it for a month or two, then stop for a week, and then try another round, if desired.

This is a convenient way to take ginseng, and the amount of alcohol you take in is actually quite small. You can remove most of the alcohol by simmering the tincture in a little water for fifteen-twenty minutes. Be careful of the evaporating alcohol—it is very flammable.

GINSENG SUPPLEMENTS

If you don't want to go to the trouble of making your own ginseng tinctures or buying whole roots and making tea, there are some excellent supplements on the market. Look for supplements that are standardized for ginsenosides, the primary active ingredient in ginseng. Some products on the market have been found not to contain any measurable ginsenosides, so buying herbal products guaranteed to contain a specific amount of ginsenosides is a good way to make sure you are getting your money's worth. Ginseng tinctures manufactured in North America are also a good value, because alcohol extracts the activity well and has a stabilizing effect on the ginsenosides. Tincture-making utilizes a cold extraction process, and it is known that heat and acid break them down.

Even powdered extracts, which are the most common kind of extracts found in capsules and tablets, quickly absorb moisture with

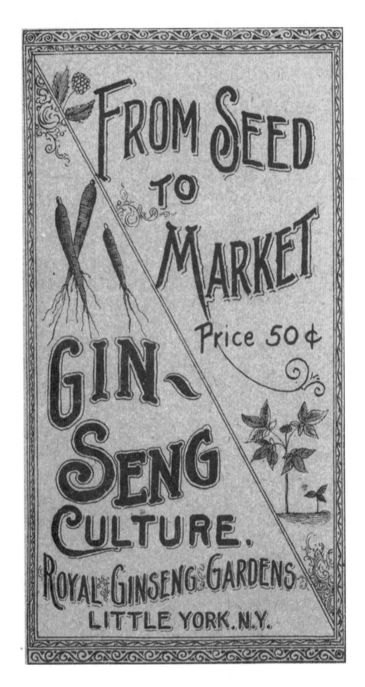

A 1902 pamphlet on ginseng growing from
the Royal Ginseng Gardens, Little York, New York

subsequent reductions in ginsenosides (Choi et al, 1984). It is important to use up a bottle of ginseng capsules or tablets within a year of purchase for maximum effectiveness. Make sure to check the "pull date" on any ginseng product. Better still, a manufacture date will tell you how long it has been on the shelf. If there is neither of these vital statistics on the bottle, it is better to avoid the product. Call the manufacturer if in doubt.

The ginsenosides in ginseng are reasonably stable, but they do break down over time. For instance, after a storage period of three years, the ginsenoside content of white ginseng decreased by 27% and of red ginseng, 12%, and exposure to moisture greatly speeded the process (Noh et al, 1983). Other quality factors such as the ratio of various ginsenosides also decline (Choi et al, 1983). The traditional processing that creates red ginseng is thought to help preserve its activity. Freeze-drying preserves the ginsenosides better than any other drying method, followed by careful air-drying (Zhang, 1983).

QUALITY GUIDELINES

As with most herbs, there are many factors that go into the making of a quality ginseng product. These include the following:

> Growing conditions, such as the nutritional status of the soil
> Time of year in which the roots are harvested
. > Drying method
> Length of storage before they are processed
> Form of the product, whether tincture, tablet, or tea
> Standardized to ginsenosides or not?

Another crucial factor is the honesty and care of the manufacturer. For instance, it has been rumored that some manufacturers use ginseng that has already had the ginsenosides removed (for use in other products) to make capsules and tablets. A trained herbalist often can estimate the quality of a ginseng root by taste, appearance, and smell, but when the herb has already been made into a tablet, especially when it is blended with vitamins, minerals, and other nutritional supplements, it is difficult to judge it. In a 1995 *Consumer Reports* review of herbal products, the editors report on a study the magazine commissioned on a sampling of commercial ginseng products. They had ten nationally-distributed ginseng products tested for ginsenoside content and found a high variability among them. Several had nearly insignificant amounts of ginsenosides, almost as if they contained "spent" ginseng. The other products ranged from 2-7.5% ginsenosides.

WHO SHOULDN'T TAKE GINSENG — SIDE EFFECTS AND CAUTIONS

Panax ginseng is a safe herb when used with knowledge and with moderation. It has very low acute toxicity—even the lethal dose of the purified ginsenosides given orally to mice is five grams/kilogram of body weight. If humans were as sensitive to the purified ginsenosides as mice, a corresponding lethal dose would be about three-hundred grams, nearly three-quarters of a pound! Because ginseng products have been used by millions of people for at least three-thousand years, it is safe to assume that toxicity of whole root and leaf products is not a major problem. Chronic exposure also was tested in dogs. A special standardized ginseng extract (G115) was given orally up to 15 mg/kg/ day for ninety days. No side effects were noted, and blood and tissue samples from the liver and other organs were normal (Hess et al, 1983).

However, ginseng is not appropriate for everyone. Because reports of its effects on blood pressure are contradictory—it raises blood pressure at low doses and may lower it at higher doses, but some studies find different effects—it is not a good idea to take a tonic course of ginseng if you suffer from high blood pressure, at least, not unless you are under careful medical supervision, especially a practitioner trained in Chinese medicine. More broadly, *Panax ginseng*, especially red, is a heating yang tonic, so it is not appropriate for people who are already "overheated," with symptoms such as headaches, palpitations, or insomnia. Indeed, it can bring on those symptoms in some people. It is not a good idea for people who have a strong pulse, who are overweight, or who have various "heat" conditions, such as asthma, inflammation, infections, colds, flu, or an acute infectious disease accompanied by fever. It can make these conditions worse (Bergner, 1992). Women of childbearing years should be careful not to take large amounts of ginseng, especially red ginseng, as it might increase estrogen levels and possibly affect menstrual cycles. Pregnant women should be cautious when using ginseng for the same reason. (On the other hand, post-menopausal women may benefit from ginseng's possible estrogenic effects).

Ginseng is thought of as a sympathetic nervous system stimulant by

Chinese researchers (Lou et al, 1989). One group reports two cases of visual disturbances possibly related to overstimulation of the sympathetic (adrenergic) nerves due to an overdose of ginseng. The two patients reported abnormal iris dilation, disturbance in accommodation, as well as dizziness and semiconsciousness.

If ginseng does increase sympathetic tone, it might be best to avoid ginseng intake (especially red ginseng) during times of acute stress, anxiety, nervousness, or sleeplessness. Stephen Fulder, author of the respected *The Tao of Medicine*, related this cautionary view of the herb:

> *In general, people who are highly energetic, nervous, tense, hysteric, manic or schizophrenic should not take ginseng.*

In one 28-year-old patient, an inflammation of arteries of the brain was noted, after she used large quantities of an alcoholic extract of ginseng (Ryu & Chien, 1995).

Because ginseng can stimulate the production of anti-diuretic hormone and markedly reduce urinary output in animals, consult a TCM practitioner if you have trouble with water-retention or edema, especially associated with high blood pressure.

At this time, we should clear up some misconceptions about "ginseng abuse syndrome." Siegel (1979) first reported this syndrome in people who took large amounts of ginseng. It consisted of elevated blood pressure, nervousness, insomnia, skin eruptions, and diarrhea in 10% of 133 ginseng users. However, many of those who experienced the symptoms were also users of great amounts of caffeine. In fact, some commentators have written that it should be renamed "ginseng-caffeine-abuse syndrome." Some of the people who experienced these symptoms were also taking large amounts of ginseng—15 grams of powdered ginseng capsules a day, which works out to 30 (500 mg) capsules a day! As the author of the original study recently told a reporter, "Our interest is only to try to understand why people were coming into our emergency rooms with problems...the problem is theirs. I don't think it is ginseng's at all" (Blumenthal, 1991).

Another, more recent controversy surrounded Eleuthero (Siberian ginseng). It was reported (Koren & Randor et al, 1990) that women who were taking Siberian ginseng while they were pregnant gave birth to babies that showed signs of excess male characteristics (androgenization). However, upon closer study, it turned out that the supplement the women thought was eleuthero was actually an unrelated herb, *Periploca sepium* Bunge, "Chinese silk vine." Even this herb does not seem to cause androgenatization in animals, though, so the actual cause of the problem, while it is clearly not eleuthero, remains a mystery (Waller et al, 1992).

It is easy to dismiss these negative reports in the medical literature, for they have obvious scientific faults. But that doesn't mean that we should not be careful about potentially potent herbs such as ginseng. As we have noted, too much ginseng, especially red ginseng, can be overstimulating and probably should be avoided by people who have high blood pressure. As for pregnant women, the disturbing factor is not that Siberian ginseng caused a problem in their infants—it clearly didn't—but that they thought they had bought eleuthero or Siberian ginseng and were actually taking Chinese silk vine. That's one reason why we should buy our herbal products from reputable suppliers, who know what they are buying, where it comes from, and how it is harvested. For a list of suppliers, see the Resource Section.

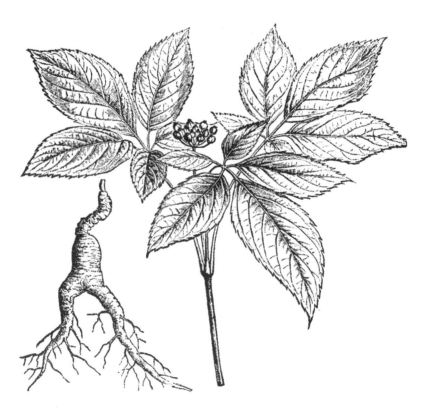

Panax quinquefolius from *Medical Botany* by W. Woodville, 1742

Summary of Noted Side Effects

(when inappropriately used based on constitutional type or condition, or when the dose is too high, or it is taken for too long)

➤ Irritability, excitation (tincture)
➤ Intoxication with spots before the eyes, headache, dizziness
➤ Spontaneous bleeding is said to be a characteristic sign of ginseng intoxication (Chang & But, 1986)
➤ Breathlessness, chest discomfort, abdominal distention (in excess-type individuals)
➤ Newborns were intoxicated by a tea from 0.3-0.6 grams of ginseng; one is reported to have died (Chang & But, 1986)
➤ Prolonged use of more than 300 mg of the powder might lead to insomnia, depression, headache, heart palpitations, hypertension, diminished sexual function, and weight loss (Chang & But, 1986)

Summary of Cautions for Ginseng Use

Avoid red ginseng use if you have the following conditions or symptoms:

➤ High blood pressure
➤ Irritability, nervousness
➤ Emotional or psychological imbalances
➤ Headaches, palpitations, or insomnia and feel hot or have a very strong pulse
➤ Asthma
➤ Inflammation
➤ Infections, colds, flu, or any acute infectious diseases accompanied by fever
➤ During pregnancy, it is best to avoid Tienqi ginseng or red ginseng; moderate use of American ginseng should be no problem for most women

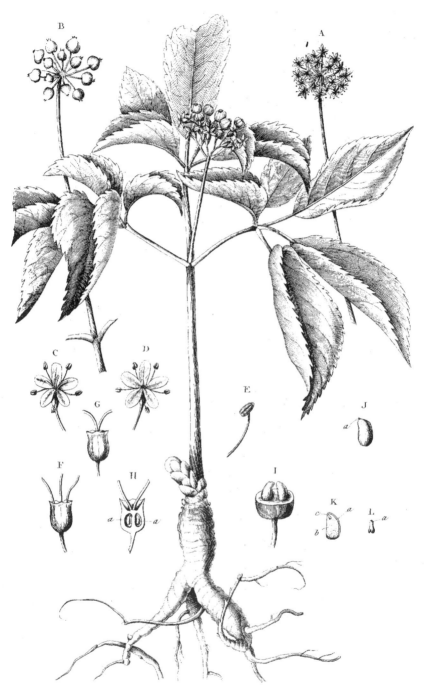

Panax quinquefolius from *An Illustrated Flora of the Northern U.S., Canada, and the British Possessions* by Britton & Brown, 1897

PART THREE

Profiles of Ginsengs & Related Herbs

PANAX GINSENG, RED

CHINESE NAME: Ren shen (also called Hong shen)
LATIN NAME: *Panax ginseng*
ENERGY/PROPERTIES: sweet, mild, bitter, warm
CHANNELS ENTERED: Lung, Spleen
DOSAGE: 1-9 g of root powder, or an equivalent amount of extract; products standardized to 4-5% ginsenosides are available, and some companies claim that a ratio of Rg1 to Rb1 of 1:2 is desirable, but this has not been well-substantiated by controlled studies. The dosage recommended by the German Kommission E (Blumenthal, 1996) is 1-2 g of the powdered herb or equivalent product for up to two 2-month periods. The French *Bulletin Officiel* No. 90/22 bis recommends a dose not to exceed 2 grams of powder/day, for not longer than 3 months.

Red ginseng is warmer in nature and more stimulating than white ginseng, and red Korean ginseng is the most stimulating ginseng of all. Red Chinese ginseng is not as strong or as stimulating as Korean, but it has a similar energy and is less expensive.

All ginseng roots, when peeled, are white. Ginseng turns red from the way it is processed. It is steamed slowly, which makes it very hard, and then dried. Sometimes it is soaked with honey or wine first, which makes it more suitable for treating yin deficiency. The steaming process causes a fundamental change in the steroids (ginsenosides) in the ginseng root, and it makes it much more stimulating.

Red ginseng is sometimes used for people who have strong constitutions and want more energy—it is used often in energy, weight-lifting, and sports formulas. However, this is not a balanced way of using ginseng. It should not be used for long periods of time by people who are under forty or fifty who just want a rush (herbal speed). If you drank two or three cups of this red ginseng, you might actually get slight heart palpitations or feel anxious or overstimulated, or you might not be able to sleep.

Red Korean ginseng is said to replenish our root vitality and expel pathogens. Chinese texts also state that it can help support the fluids and structure of the lung, soothe the soul, clear the vision, stimulate digestion, and control heart palpitations.

When someone is very weak and doesn't have enough vitality, that is when the red variety can be useful. In the Chinese materia medica the use of ginseng in general, and red ginseng in particular, is indicated for people who have "collapsed Qi" with "devastated yang" (Bensky and Gamble, 1986). This type of person can feel very cold, have a low sex drive, and appear lackluster and withdrawn. It is used for the elderly and for people with serious disorders of Yang and Qi, not for a little pick-me-up. This is the older person's remedy, because it is said to increase blood circulation and sexual hormone production, such as testosterone and estrogen. The excessive use of ginseng for extended periods (more than a few weeks) can lead to imbalances even in the elderly.

Remember that red ginseng is almost always blended with other herbs in traditional formulas—spleen-tonifying herbs, like astragalus, atractylodes (*Atractylodes macrocephala* Koidz.), or fuling (*Wolfiporia cocos* [Schwein.] Ryv. & Gilbn.), or digestive-moving herbs, like ginger, cardamon (*Elettaria cardamomum* [L.] Maton), or citrus (such as orange) peel to help counteract ginseng's tendency to lead to a feeling of fullness in the chest and diaphragm if overused. Adding ginger and a little licorice (*Glycyrrhiza glabra* L.) will modify the stimulating quality.

It is also worth exploring the notion that red ginseng can "calm the spirit." How can an herb that is stimulating and heating be calming? The answer isn't in the ginseng, but in the individuals for whom ginseng is best suited. Sometimes if you feel very fatigued and run-down, you will often feel anxious as well, since being very deficient in energy can lead to anxiety. So used in the proper circumstances, ginseng will calm the spirit, stop heart palpitations, and alleviate anxiety. For overstimulated people with strong constitutions, it can actually bring those symptoms on.

SUMMARY OF MEDICAL USES IN CHINA
> ➤ Revival of dying patients, for shock and cardiac failure (used with treated aconite)
> ➤ Impotence, sexual weakness
> ➤ Mental fatigue
> ➤ Long-term debility with tiredness and sleeping problems

➤ Mild diabetes to reduce blood glucose levels (possible 40-50 mg/dl reduction within 2 weeks); for moderate to severe diabetes, ginseng is used in conjunction with insulin (Chang & But, 1986)
➤ Digestive weakness and poor assimilation, especially in the elderly, to increase appetite
➤ With cancer patients to improve appetite and support immune function
➤ Asthma, shortness of breath
➤ Patients with psychological disturbances

SUMMARY OF USES
in the *Pharmacopeia of the People's Republic of China* (Tu, 1988):
INDICATIONS: Prostration with impending collapse marked by cold limbs and faint pulse, to benefit the *spleen* and the *lung,* to preserve the production of body fluid, and to calm the nerves.

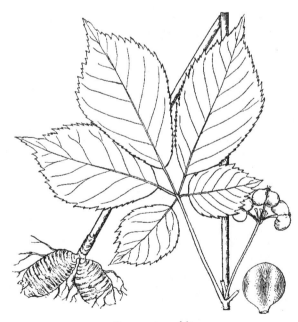

Panax quinquefolius
from *Medical Botany of North America* by L. Johnson, 1884

PANAX GINSENG, WHITE

CHINESE NAME: Ren shen, Sheng shai shen
LATIN NAME: *Panax ginseng*
ENERGY/PROPERTIES: sweet, slightly bitter, slightly warm
CHANNELS ENTERED: Lung, Spleen
DOSAGE: 1-9 g

Chinese white ginseng, which is simply the fresh-dried cultivated root of *P. ginseng,* is the mildest of the Asian ginsengs. White Chinese ginseng is more yin than red Chinese or Korean ginseng, but less of a yin tonic than American ginseng. In China, fresh-dried white ginseng is sometimes used as a substitute for American ginseng, because of its similar properties.

Like red ginseng, white ginseng is almost always used in combination with other herbs. When someone is weak and ill, he or she may be given ginseng (with ginger or licorice) to support the Qi, so that the body is strong enough to withstand the effects of stronger specific herbs. The best white ginseng is a very pale yellow.

See the next section for more specific information on how White Chinese ginseng is used.

TABLE 3
THE TRADITIONAL USES OF AMERICAN GINSENG IN NORTH AMERICA

Penobscots	promoting female fertility
Iroquois	decoction of the roots as a panacea, for fainting spells, used for laziness and as a stimulant, for tuberculosis, as a strengthener of the mental powers, eye medicine
Mohawks	an ordinary remedy for intermittent fever
Cherokees	headaches, cramps, "female troubles," analgesic, weakness of the womb and nervous affections, tonic and expectorant, for "thrush," as an expectorant, for short-windedness, any severe illness; a cure when others have failed; universal remedy for children and adults, decoction to stop vomiting; for rheumatism, for a bad appetite, for tapeworms, wash for eyes
Creeks	to keep ghosts away, to induce sweating, reduce fever, croup in children, infusion for shortness of breath, hoarse coughing, mixed with ginger and alcohol to produce sweat; to stop bleeding from cuts
Houmas	boiled roots used to stop vomiting and with whiskey to ease rheumatism
Menominees	tonic and strengtheners of mental powers
Meskwakis	universal remedy; as a seasoner to add power to other medicines; mixed with other herbs for use as a love potion
Pottawatomis	pounded root was used as a poultice to cure earache and soaked then pounded as a wash for sore eyes; to mask unpleasant tastes

[Drawn from Vogel, 1970; Moerman, 1986]

AMERICAN GINSENG

CHINESE NAME: Xi yang shen
LATIN NAME: *Panax quinquefolius*
ENERGY/PROPERTIES: sweet, slightly bitter, neutral, cool
CHANNELS ENTERED: Lung, Stomach/Spleen
DOSAGE: 3-9 g

It is often difficult to distinguish what impact exposure to European culture had on the uses by Native American Indians of indigenous plants, including American ginseng. Some of the uses reported from various tribes are unusually close to Chinese uses, leading one to at least consider a cultural influence, East to West. It is always of interest to compare the use of specific medicinal plants from the same genus where they occur in both North America and Asia (disjunct species; see Foster & Chongxi, 1992). The preceding table summarizes the uses of American ginseng in north America by indigenous people.

Due in part to the intense desire of the Chinese for wild American roots in the early days of this country and the good price that it brought from its export, ginseng became a folk-remedy among rural people in the Eastern United States in its own right. American ginseng never did achieve much support from American medical practitioners of the 18th, 19th, and early 20th centuries. It was thought to be nothing more than a mild digestive tonic and a gentle stimulant with antispasmodic properties (Griffith, 1847), or a sweetener for medicines, similar in taste to licorice (Coxe, 1830). Though a Dr. Fothergill reports (Bigelow, 1817) that "in tedious chronic coughs, incident to people in years, a decoction of it has been of service." An interesting connection can be made between this use by an American doctor of the very early 19th century and the Chinese use of American ginseng for "weak Lung Qi." Benjamin Barton Smith (1810), one of the first extensive writers on the American native medicinal plants, said that ginseng is to be classed with the stimulants, and that "If it were not a native of our woods, it is probable that we should import it, as we do the teas of China and Japan, at a high price." American ginseng was official in the U.S. Pharmacopeia from 1840-1870 only (Gathercoal & Youngkin, 1942). In the U.S. National Dispensatory, 24th edition (Osol & Farrar, 1947), which is a semi-official commentary on the official drugs of the pharmacopeia plus other popularly-used medicines of the day, the most enthusiasm the authors could manage is "It is little more than a demulcent, and in this country is rarely employed as a medicine."

The eclectic doctors were a school of medically-trained physicians who believed that herbal medicine was superior and less harmful than synthetic drugs and toxic metals. They flourished from the late 1800s to the 1930s and at one point operated numerous medical institutions and published respected medical journals. A number of excellent texts emerged from this period, and herbalists today still use the Eclectic medical literature as an important source of information about the therapeutic uses of medicinal plants. The most complete compilation of Eclectic medical uses of herbs can be found in the Felter & Lloyd (1898) revision of the *King's American Dispensatory*. It is a commonly-consulted work, especially on native American medicinal plants. The best clinical information on these plants comes from the works of the Eclectics. The Eclectics recommended American ginseng as a mild tonic and stimulant, "Useful in loss of appetite, slight nervous debility, and weak stomach." Felter & Lloyd described it as "a very important remedy in nervous dyspepsia, and in mental exhaustion from over-work" (neurasthenia). They also recommended it in an infusion (2-4 ounces/dose) or as a powder (4 grams/dose) for relieving asthma, atonic laryngitis, and bronchitis.

American ginseng is the most balanced of the *Panax* ginsengs. It is both a yin and a yang tonic. A commercial root will taste fairly bland and a little sweet, but if you get to taste a good wild root, it will be at first sweet and then have a pleasant bitter flavor, which is characteristic of good ginseng. The woods-grown American roots are more nourishing to the Yin (supports the adrenals, regulates the basic metabolism, and increases fluids) for longer term use. I tend to use it myself when I am feeling rundown. It is traditionally used to nourish Yin, clear heat, increase salivation, and supplement and moisten the lungs.

I consider American ginseng, especially the wild but also woods-grown, to be very beneficial for overstressed, overworked, adrenal-weak Americans. While red ginseng is too stimulating and heating for most healthy people under age fifty, at least for long-term use, American ginseng can be very useful. Because it is more cooling than these other kinds of ginsengs, it can be appropriate for younger, hotter, stressed individuals.

Wild ginseng is expensive, so woods-grown is the best option for most people. Look for roots that are hard, fibrous, and slightly bitter. Cultivated American ginseng is less expensive, but also not as effective as the other two. Organically-cultivated roots are just now becoming available, but make sure they are certified organically-grown. Chinese white is the least expensive of all.

PRINCE'S GINSENG

CHINESE NAME: Tai zi shen
LATIN NAME: *Pseudostellaria heterophylla*
ENERGY/PROPERTIES: sweet, slightly bitter, neutral
CHANNELS ENTERED: Lung, Spleen
DOSAGE: 9-30 g.

Prince's ginseng is a useful energy (Qi) tonic that is, nevertheless, unrelated botanically to ginseng. It is actually in the carnation family. It is a small root from a Chinese plant and is used as a general tonic. Prince's ginseng is not as stimulating as the *Panax* ginsengs, especially the red ginseng. Like American ginseng (*Panax quinquefolius*), it stimulates the production of body fluids, tonifying the Qi.

If you feel lethargic, weak, or rundown, or one of your organs is not working efficiently due to lack of energy, that is called Qi deficiency. If your digestion is not working efficiently, this is what is called in Chinese medicine spleen Qi deficiency—in other words, digestive energy deficiency. Prince's ginseng can actually increase your digestive powers, so you can better digest and assimilate food. Most of our energy comes from food, and if our digestive system is not strong enough to convert food into energy, then we have to draw on our reserve energy. The longer we have to draw on our reserves, the more quickly we age, and that's when adrenal fatigue, chronic fatigue syndrome, and all of these types of chronic ailments take place—when we don't have enough daily energy to supply our bodies' needs and have to draw from our reserves.

Recent research from the Chinese University of Hong Kong suggests that Prince's ginseng may have immune benefits. In animal studies, it has both immune-stimulating and anti-tumor effects (Wong et al, 1994). It stimulates production of natural killer cells and T cells and also tumor necrosis factor, which helps fight tumors.

Another advantage of Prince's ginseng is that it is substantially cheaper than *Panax ginseng*. It is a very common wild plant in China, and most of it is harvested from the wild. It is also used for mental fatigue, loss of appetite, and chronic illnesses.

I recommend that tonics be used for at least a month or two to give them a fair trial, so you might want to try Prince's ginseng for a few weeks. Remember that herbs are not like drugs. They work more slowly, behind the scenes, to restore balance and harmony. They supply materials our bodies need, but they are not really flogging and whipping our adrenals into activity like a cup of coffee would. Coffee may make you feel great for a while, but then your energy will dwindle, because basically when you stimulate the body processes when you don't have the actual energy within yourself, then eventually you are going to create illness and weaken your natural energy.

You can take Prince's ginseng as a food, in soups or stews, for up to two years. Look for thick, moist, yellowish-white roots without small rootlets.

TIENQI GINSENG

CHINESE NAME: Sanqi, or Tienqi
LATIN NAME: *Panax notoginseng*; also known as *Panax pseudoginseng*
ENERGY/PROPERTIES: sweet, slightly bitter, warm
CHANNELS ENTERED: Liver, Stomach, Large Intestine
DOSAGE: 3-9 g/day as whole root in decoction; 1-1.5 g 3 x daily as a powder; a "course" is 4 weeks, take 1-12 courses as needed with a 3-day break between (Chang & But, 1986).

In this book we have several herbs that are unrelated to the true ginsengs, yet which act similarly as energy tonics. Tienqi ginseng is the converse: it is botanically related to ginseng—it is a true *Panax*—but it is not used as a general energy tonic. Rather, it is used primarily to move blood and reduce pain—in China it is the herb of choice for traumatic injuries. In Chinese medicine it is always thought that if there is pain or swelling, it is due to stagnant blood. Tienqi is used—externally or internally—for moving the blood, reducing the pain, and for its warming properties. Moreover, it is very famous as an astringent for controlling bleeding.

The herb is also a specific tonic to the heart. In recent years, its cardiac effects have been increasingly studied. Animal studies suggest that *Panax notoginseng* can dilate coronary arteries (Lei and Chiou, 1986) and help the heart muscle recover from injury due to lack of oxygen (ischemia). In a clinical study of 16 patients with angina, the pain was significantly reduced in 15 of those studied (Bensky and Gamble, 1986). This particular ginseng has also been shown to have anti-inflammatory and analgesic (pain-killing) effects in animals (Wang et al, 1994), as well as a negative chronotropic (slows heart-beat) and inotropic (affects heartbeat) effect, and a selective vasodilating effect on coronary arteries (Huang, 1993), increasing blood flow, while decreasing the heart rate (Hu et al, 1992). It also reduces the tendency of blood to clot (Shi et al, 1990). So it can be a beneficial herb to use, under medical supervision and guidance of a TCM practitioner, if you have heart disease.

The general dose is 3-9 grams per day. For a decoction, you take the herb and place it in about five times as much water. If you start with one ounce of the herb, you add it to five ounces of water, and then boil or simmer it over low heat for about forty-five minutes.

CAUTIONS AND CONTRAINDICATIONS

Do not exceed recommended dose; adverse effects on the heart's conduction system have been noted in doses over 5 grams.

Some sensitive individuals might experience such symptoms as nausea, vomiting, hemoptysis, epistaxis, gingival bleeding, menorrhagia; reduce dose or discontinue if these symptoms occur.

SUMMARY OF USE IN CHINA (*Under medical supervision only*)
- ➤ To relieve pain of angina pectoris (dilates coronary arteries, increases flow to heart muscle); dose, 1 gram 3 x daily
- ➤ To stop pain and promote healing in traumatic injury
- ➤ To stop bleeding of hemorrhages
- ➤ Hemoptysis, spitting of blood from lungs (6-9 grams of herb powder is used 2-3 x daily for 5-7 days until bleeding stops)
- ➤ Hematuria, blood in the urine (1-1.5 grams every 4-8 hours until bleeding is stopped)
- ➤ For excessive loss of blood and anemia (when the herb is processed or "cured") *From Chang & But* (1986)

Zhu Je Ginseng

Chinese name: Zhujieshen, Zhuzishen
Latin name: *Panax japonicus* C.A. Meyer, *P. japonicus* var. *major*
Energy/Properties: bitter
Channels entered: Stomach/Spleen
Dosage: see below

Zhujeshen ginseng is called Tikusetuninzin in Japan. It is used as a substitute for *Panax ginseng*. The herb is thought to strengthen the stomach and digestion, eliminating excess phlegm. Medically it is recommended for a feeling of fullness, distention, or obstruction in the abdomen. Practitioners of TCM use it for treating accumulation of fluid around the heart, to ease heart palpitations, nausea and vomiting, and to increase appetite in people with anorexia (Hsu, 1986).

The Chinese Pharmacopeia (English Edition, 1988) gives the following actions and indications:

> **Action:** to strengthen the constitution, to eliminate blood stasis and relieve pain, to arrest bleeding, and to promote expectoration.
> **Indications:** General weakness after disease; consumptive cough with hemoptysis, cough with profuse sputum; traumatic injuries.
> **Dose:** 6-9 grams

Zhuzishen, *P. japonicus* var. *major* is also official.
> **Action:** To nourish Yin and replenish the lung, to promote the flow of Qi in collaterals, and to arrest bleeding.
> **Indications:** Deficiency of both Qi and Yin characterized by fever and thirst, cough in consumptive diseases, traumatic injuries, joint pain; hemoptysis, hematemesis, traumatic bleeding.
> **Dose:** 3-9 grams

ELEUTHERO (SIBERIAN GINSENG)

CHINESE NAME: Ciwujia
LATIN NAME: *Eleutherococcus senticosus*
ENERGY/PROPERTIES: acrid, warm
CHANNELS ENTERED: Kidney, Lung, Spleen
DOSAGE: 5-15 g

Eleuthero is more neutral than the *Panax* ginsengs; it is used less for digestion and more for its anti-stress, glandular/adrenal system effects; it also supports immunity. In general, eleuthero can be taken for longer periods than *Panax*, without being concerned about estrogenic and testosterone-inducing effects. It is generally not as stimulating.

Eleuthero is good for people who just want a tonic, a pick me up, to normalize body functions. It is a remarkable adaptogen, as documented earlier in this book, and a useful herb to take if you are undergoing stress or need to perform under difficult conditions. The herb is also widely used by athletes to increase performance and endurance and to help recover more quickly from a strenuous workout. It is known to help muscles utilize oxygen and energy stores more efficiently.

Eleuthero can be taken in tea, tincture, or capsule form. I prefer tea or tincture for a period of 2 or 3 months—up to 8 months. It does affect the pituitary gland and help regulate all the hormonal functions of the body. The dose of the tincture is 2 droppers at a time, morning and evening. If you are recovering from illness, or if your energy is in a state of collapse, ginseng is preferable. If you are just under stress, eleuthero is preferred.

The herb is official in *The Chinese Pharmacopeia* (English Edition, 1988):

ACTIONS: To reinforce Qi, to invigorate the function of the Spleen and the Kidney, and to calm the nerves.

INDICATIONS: Hypofunction of the Spleen and the Kidney marked by general weakness, lassitude, anorexia, aching of the loins and knees; insomnia and dream-disturbed sleep.

DOSE: 9-27 grams.

CODONOPSIS ROOT (FALSE GINSENG)

CHINESE NAME: Dang Shen
LATIN NAME: *Codonopsis pilosula*
ENERGY/PROPERTIES: sweet, neutral
CHANNELS ENTERED: Lung, Spleen
DOSAGE: 9-30g.

Codonopsis, or *dang shen*, is often used as a milder, less stimulating, and less expensive ginseng. It is used in food, to strengthen digestion, increase assimilation of nutrients, and tone the "middle burner," which in Chinese medicine includes the stomach and the Spleen system (pancreas and small intestine). It is often used when there is a lack of appetite, fatigue, tired limbs, or diarrhea (Bensky and Gamble, 1986). It has been studied for its ulcer-protective properties (Li et al, 1987). Like ginseng, it also tonifies the lungs and has been used clinically to treat bronchitis (Feng and Song, 1985).

The cardiovascular effects of codonopsis have been fairly well studied. In one study (Wang and Zhu, 1990) 24 patients with angina (chest pains that often occur with coronary heart disease) were given 20 grams of codonopsis three times a day for seven days. Ten controls were given aspirin, which is known to reduce the tendency of blood to clot and is a standard treatment for heart disease patients. Like aspirin, codonopsis reduced the clotting factors thromboxane A_2 and prostacyclin. In China, codonopsis is sometimes administered to heart disease patients in combination with astragalus, an immune-boosting herb (Liao et al, 1988) and has been shown to reduce the immunosuppressive effects of radiation on cancer patients (Zneg et al, 1992). It may also lower blood pressure (Bensky and Gamble, 1986).

Dang shen is an important herb for improving digestive power and increasing overall energy. If you are feeling rundown and experiencing weak digestion, you might benefit from a decoction of codonopsis. In Traditional Chinese Medicine (TCM), dang shen is used in place of ginseng to tonify the Qi of the spleen and lungs, whereas ginseng is used for the more serious disorder of collapsed Qi with "devastated yang," according to *Chinese Materia Medica*, by Bensky and Gamble (1986). It is better for more normal kinds of fatigue and everyday stress.

Look for thick, firm, tight-skinned roots. Use one or one-and-a-half roots per day, with two cups of water, and boil down until you get one cup; then add fresh grated ginger to taste. Drink one cup in the morning and one in the evening. You can also add some codonopsis root into a stew or a soup. It is an ingredient in many Chinese formulas.

DANG GUI

CHINESE NAME: Dang gui (also called Tang Kwai, Dong Quai)
LATIN NAME: *Angelica sinensis, A. acutiloba* (in Japan)
ENERGY/PROPERTIES: sweet, acrid; warm
CHANNELS ENTERED: Heart, Liver, Spleen
DOSAGE: 9-15g.

The herb dang gui is perhaps the most widely-used herb in the world, and it is certainly the most popular Chinese herb (Huang, 1993). That is because many of the approximately one-half billion Chinese women, as well as millions of Japanese women, and women from many other Asian countries, use the herb in their daily lives as an all-around tonic and to strengthen their reproductive organs and regulate their menstrual cycle. If a Chinese or Asian woman feels run-down or tired, especially if related to her monthly cycle, she might depend on dang gui in a soup or other recipe to give her an energy boost. Although it has been called "women's ginseng," it is not just for women. The herb is commonly prescribed by herbalists and acupuncturists in herb prescriptions for both men and women. Its main action is to "build and regulate the blood." Dang gui is known to have coumarins, chemical compounds that thin the blood, and is reported to contain a high amount of vitamin B12, a nutrient that is essential

DANG GUI CHICKEN OR VEGETABLE SOUP RECIPE

2 tblsp olive oil	2 tblsp miso, dissolved in warm water
1 green pepper, chopped	5 cups Dang gui tea
1 carrot, thinly sliced	3 cloves garlic, minced
1 onion, thinly sliced	1 tsp fresh ginger
1/4 head green cabbage, thinly sliced	1/4 tsp oregano
2 stalks celery, thinly sliced	1/2 tsp basil
1 cup mushrooms, thinly sliced	1/2 tsp tamari
1 cake tofu, diced (or 1 lb chicken)	1/4 tsp salt

Sauté the vegetables in the olive oil until tender. Add the ginger, garlic, and spices and cook 2 minutes more. Add the tofu (or chicken), miso, and Dang gui tea, and simmer gently for 30-45 minutes. Garnish with thinly sliced green onions.

for the production of red blood cells, as well as a high-molecular weight polysaccharide that may stimulate the blood-producing process in the bone marrow.

In markets and grocery stores throughout China, as well as in Chinatowns throughout the world, it is common to see a display of dang gui crowns, with their strong celery-like aroma. These crowns are purchased by the pound for use in many kinds of recipes.

One famous recipe is given on the preceding page.

The confusion about dang gui is related to its principal activity. First of all, as far as is known presently, it does not affect the hormones. For instance, several studies have stated that dang gui does not appear to have an estrogenic effect. There are no clinical or laboratory studies available from China or any other country that report this activity, as can be found in a search of Medline, Biosis, Chemical Abstracts, or other primary references (Chang & But, 1986; Huang, 1993; Tang & Eisenbrand, 1992; Mei et al, 1991). Numerous published reports of animal studies performed in China have found that dang gui water extracts and alcoholic extracts administered orally or by injections do have the following effects:

➤ Relaxing or stimulating effect on the smooth muscle of the uterus (tincture is more relaxing, tea is more stimulating), increasing blood flow, local nutrition and DNA synthesis, stimulating growth
➤ Lower blood pressure, dilate the coronary vessels and increase coronary flow, inhibit the formation of blood clots; the heart muscle seems to use less oxygen
➤ Preventative effect on cardiovascular disease (atherosclerosis)
➤ Antihistamine, anti-inflammatory, antibody-inhibitory activity
➤ Relax the bronchial tree, demonstrating an anti-asthmatic effect
➤ Prevent platelet aggregation, reduce plasma fibrinogen, decrease blood viscosity, prolonging the coagulation time of blood
➤ Extracts increase colony-stimulating factors (CSF) in spleen cells of healthy mice (Chen & Gao, 1994)
➤ Protective effect on the liver
➤ Anti-tumor effect of low-molecular weight polysaccharide (Choy et al, 1994)
➤ Mild sedative effect
➤ Mild antibiotic effect

[Summarized from Chang & But, 1986, Bensky & Gamble, 1986, Mei et al, 1991; Shi, 1995]

What relevance these studies have in determining how dang gui works in the human system is open to debate. In Chinese hospitals and clinical practice, dang gui extracts are commonly used in teas and patent formulas in the form of syrups, alcoholic extracts, candy, tablets, and capsules. They are also commonly administered by injection to various parts of the body, often into acupuncture points to reduce pain, swelling, and other symptoms and promote healing in arthritis, skin diseases, chronic obstructive pulmonary disease (COPD), and numerous other conditions.

A number of clinical reports (uncontrolled studies) have been translated from Chinese and are briefly summarized below.

➤ Good therapeutic effects in relieving symptoms of PMS (dysmenorrhea, amenorrhea, breast tenderness, cramps, hot flashes, constipation, and dizziness); promotes smooth blood flow, reducing inflammation or irritation
➤ Symptoms of pelvic inflammatory disease (PID) were benefited
➤ Helps reverse sterility
➤ Calms the fetus
➤ Beneficial effects on kidney function and kidney disease
➤ Helped patients with chronic bronchitis complicated with emphysema, chronic obstructive pulmonary disease, or pulmonary heart disease (in the early stages); increased forced expiratory volume
➤ Good results in treating anemia, especially when combined with white peony, *Paeonia alba*, or astragalus, *Astragalus membranaceous*.
➤ Beneficial effects were noted on patients with hepatitis and cirrhosis
[Summarized from Chang & But; 1986, Huang, 1993; Mei et al, 1991]

CAUTIONS:

Because of the stimulating effect on the uterus reported from dang gui extracts, it is wise to avoid its use in cases of endometriosis. Because of its coumarin content, which can thin the blood and promote bleeding (blood-moving effect), and its possible uterine-stimulating effect, it is best to avoid its use during pregnancy and with people who have a tendency to bleed too much. Research has also been reported on the ability of dang gui extracts to lower the prothrombin time (PT) in rabbits when given with the common blood-thinning drug warfarin. The researchers warn against the use of dang gui with people who are taking blood-thinning medications (Lo, 1995).

The tea and tincture have moderately low acute toxicity, but it is wise to follow the dosage instructions on products and not to exceed the traditional dose of the bulk herb in teas, about 3-15 grams (Bensky & Gamble, 1986).

The traditional contraindications include a caution against the use of dang gui with people who have diarrhea or chronic water-retention due to weakened digestive function. People who have weakened adrenal function with signs of chronic infection, headaches, night sweats, or skin rashes should not use the herb.

SUMMARY OF USES

The most common use of dang gui in the west is for strengthening the female reproductive organs, either during the reproductive years or at the time of menopause. It may be appropriate well after the change of life. The herb is included in many products that are designed to help ease the symptoms of PMS, especially menstrual blood flow that is slow or stuck. Avoid its use when the flow is too profuse.

Dang gui is commonly recommended for men and women who have "blood deficiency." This is more comprehensive than simple anemia. In traditional medicine, blood deficiency is a condition brought on by weak digestion (the blood is thought to originate from the food, with the aid of the digestive system), stress, poor diet, and poor health habits in general. Symptoms of blood deficiency include fatigue; pale cheeks, lips and tongue; low blood pressure; depression; mental confusion; dizziness (especially upon rising quickly); and scanty or absent menstrual flow.

If you suspect you might be blood deficient, it is often wise to consult with a trained herbalist or practitioner of Traditional Chinese Medicine. Dang gui can be used as a supplement, along with Chinese peony, in tea or tablet form. Be sure to add plenty of fresh green vegetables (chard, kale, beet greens) to the diet. Non-vegetarians can use small portions of red meat several times a week. A natural herbal, food-based iron system might also help. Avoid mineral supplements that contain medium to high concentrations of iron without consulting a qualified health practitioner or physician, as this can lead to undesirable side effects.

GLEHNIA ROOT

CHINESE NAME: Sha Shen
LATIN NAME: *Glehnia littoralis* Fr. Schmidt ex Miq.
ENERGY/PROPERTIES: mildly sweet, bland; cool
CHANNELS ENTERED: Lung, Spleen/Stomach
DOSAGE: 9-15g.

Glehnia root is another important energy tonic. In Chinese medicine it is known primarily as a yin tonic rather than a yang tonic, meaning it strengthens the fluids and reserves of the body, not the active functions and heat. It is not related botanically to ginseng; rather it is from the parsley family. Unlike Chinese or Korean *Panax ginseng*, which tend to be warm and stimulating, glehnia is cooling (it has been shown to lower temperature in animal studies). Glehnia is used in many formulas to treat overheated conditions, such as rashes, arthritis, acne, or headaches. It may also have some analgesic effects.

Glehnia, like ginseng and codonopsis, enters the Lung meridian and is used to moisten the lungs, especially when there is a dry, nonproductive cough. It also enters the Stomach meridian, generating fluid (a yin characteristic) and clearing heat, so it is often used after an illness marked by fever, when a person is dry and dehydrated. It helps with the constipation that can occur in such circumstances. Conversely, since it is a cooling herb, it is contraindicated if you are feeling chilled as well as run-down.

Look for roots that are solid, long, and yellowish-white in color.

TABLE 4: ENERGY& USES OF GINSENGS & GINSENG-LIKE HERBS

Type of Ginseng	Energy/Property	Uses	Doses
Tienqi (Sanqi) ginseng *Panax notoginseng* or P. pseudoginseng	sweet, slightly bitter, warm	controls bleeding, moves blood, reduces swelling and pain, cardiotonic	3-9 gms/day
Prince's ginseng *Pseudostellaria heterophlla*	sweet, mild, bitter, warm	supports Qi, nourishes blood; mental fatigue, loss of appetite, digestive weakness, chronic illness	15-30 gms/day
Red Korean *Panax Ginseng*	sweet, mild, bitter, warm (stronger than Chinese red)	replenishes original Qi, expels evil Qi, supplements lung yin, calms spirit, "soothes the soul," increases wisdom, controls palpitations, clears vision, benefits digestion	1-9 gms/day
Red Chinese *Panax ginseng*	sweet, slightly bitter, slight warm	tonifies original Qi, for severe collapsed Qi, strengthens spleen and stomach, benefits Yin, benefits heart Qi warmer and more stimulating than Chinese white or red or American; more for yang deficient states	1-9 gms/day
White Chinese *Panax ginseng*	sweet, slightly bitter, neutral warm	more nourishing to the Yin	1-9 gms/day
Woods-grown American *Panax quinquefolium*	sweet, slightly bitter, neutral	more nourishing to the Yin; Yin deficiency with heat signs; fevers, weakness, thirst; deficient lung yin; not as strong as *Panax ginseng*	5-15 gms/day
Pearl ginseng (Zhu zi shen) *Panax major, P. repens, P. japonicus* var. *major* (Burk.) (C.Y. Wu et K.M. Feng)	bitter, mild, sweet, cold	supplements Qi, invigorates blood, used for cough and asthma	6-9 gms/day
Ginseng neck *Panax ginseng*	bitter, mild, warm	releases phlegm and fluid, nauseant; used for chest obstruction due to phlegm	3-6 gms/day
Eleuthero *Eleutherococcus senticosus*	acrid, warm	adaptogenic, supports adrenals (kidney yin and yang); regulates blood sugar, supports immune system; counteracts stress	5-15 gms/day
Glehnia *Glehnia littoralis*	sweet, bitter mild, cold	nourishes lung yin, clears deficient heat; especially for dry, unproductive coughs, dry itchy skin	6-15 gms/day

(Table 4 – Con't)

Type of Ginseng	Energy/Property	Uses	Doses
Codonopsis *Codonopsis pilosula*	sweet, neutral	tonifies digestion, strengthens Qi; fatigue, low appetite, chronic illness with painful or weak digestion, perhaps with symptoms of diarrhea, constipation, does not cause the Qi to rise and is not so heating as *Panax* sp., best for deficient heat confirmations	12-30 gms/day
Japanese Chikusetsu ginseng (Zhu-jie-shen)	cooling	strengthens stomach, disperses phlegm, sedates and tranquilizes, invigorates (antifatigue effect), protects against stess-induced ulcers, expectorant, reduces coughs	3-9 gms/day

TABLE 5: INDICATIONS FOR THE GINSENGS

Symptom/Ailment	Ginsengs	Supporting Herbs
Allergy	Asian *Panax* species	nettles
Anemia	red Chinese, codonopsis	dang gui, nettles, yellow dock
Blood pressure, high	codonopsis	garlic, hawthorn
Cholesterol, high	Asian white ginsengs	garlic
Chronic illness	wild American, woods-grown American, red, white Chinese, eleuthero	astragalus (warming, rising,) schisandra, atractylodes, poria, etc.
Constipation	codonopsis, glehnia (with dendrobium)	rhubarb
Fatigue	with no Yin deficiency: Asian ginsengs (esp. red); with Yin deficiency: pseudostellaria, American ginsengs; either case: eleuthero	astragalus, poria atractylodes
Headaches	codonopsis, eleuthero	wood betony, periwinkle, feverfew (migraines)
Heart beat, irregular, palpitations	Asian *Panax* species (especially Korean red), tienqi, glehnia	poria, hawthorn, cactus
Heavy limbs	Asian *Panax* species	atractylodes, poria
Hemorrhage	tienqi	shepherd's purse
Inflammation, deficient types	glehnia, White Chinese, American ginsengs	echinacea
Memory, poor	Asian *Panax* species	ginkgo leaf extract, gotu kola fresh plant liquid extract
Mental fatgue	Asian *Panax* species	ginkgo leaf extract, kola nut (caution, stimulating)
Mouth Sores	Glehnia, American ginsengs	propolis topically
Mucus, excess white	ginseng neck	yerba santa
Nausea	Asian *Panax* species, ginseng neck	atractylodes or pinellia, ginger
Neurasthenia	pseudostellaria	schisandra
Pain	tienqi	Roman chamomile, valerian
Painful digestion	Asian *Panax* species, codonopsis	atractylodes, ginger, poria, licorice
Rectal bleeding	tienqi	witch hazel, shepherd's purse, agrimony
Sex drive, low	Asian *Panax* species, especially red	damiana, ginger muira puama
Stress	eleuthero, pseudostellaria	schisandra, wild oat
Swellings	tienqi	mullein, calendula, St. John's wort
Weak digestion	White Asian *Panax* Species, American ginsengs	ginger, atractylodes, poria

Appendix A:
PRACTITIONER USES OF GINSENG

Michael Tierra, L.Ac.

When someone is extremely weak and in a debilitated condition, I give them 1 whole red Chinese or Korean root daily. The root should be simmered in 6 cups of water for 3-4 hours. Cook 2 cups rice in the resulting water. After cooking, chop the ginseng and add it to the rice. Sweeten with a small quantity of honey or barley syrup.

— Michael Tierra, East West Acupuncture Clinic; author, *Way of Herbs*

Ken Smith, L.Ac.

I use American ginseng, which is cooling, for tonifying the Yin and fluids. It is good for hangovers. Korean ginseng is for cold conditions, as it is a heating herb. It tonifies the Qi, especially the spleen Qi. Chinese ginseng is fairly neutral and can be used in either warm or cold conditions. I like using it in formulas, and it has the advantage of being cheaper (it can be purchased for around $40/pound). It is good to slice it before cooking, so there is more exposure to the root.

A note of caution: Some people who are strong and robust sometimes take Korean ginseng in an effort to become even stronger. This type of individual may sometimes have high blood pressure, so taking ginseng is not appropriate for them.

— Ken Smith, Ken Smith Acupuncture

Joanna Zhao, L.Ac.

In the Clinic, I use Ginseng for nourishing the kidney qi (kidney energy) and to tonify the spleen qi (spleen energy).

I use American Ginseng to help the patient who has heart qi xu (heart energy deficiency) with symptoms of palpitations, amnesia, insomnia, absentmindedness, spontaneous sweating, and cardiac pain.

Ginseng is also useful for diabetic patients to decrease the level of blood sugar. And Ginseng is useful for cancer patients, to increase the immune energy.

Ginseng is a good and useful herb, but if not used carefully, it can cause problems, For instance, if the patient is too young, Ginseng should not be used as a long-term tonifying herb. Young patients should let their bodies build up their own energy and not depend on Ginseng.

For yang deficient patients, we can use red Ginseng. For yin deficient patients, we should not use red Ginseng, because it will cause more heat.

From clinical experience, Ginseng can also be used to assist labor. Two slices of American Ginseng are double-boiled from 1 cup to 1/2 cup and drunk when the pubic bone has opened and delivery is imminent. This will make labor easier and assist delivery.

Ginseng can be used regularly by the elderly, but the dosages are very important. Only 1 to 2 slices should be used per day, boiled in water or double-boiled. The Ginseng tea needs to be drunk slowly.

Recent research shows that Ginseng can promote phagocytosis and enhance the lymphocyte blastogenesis rate. Based on this research, I have begun to use Ginseng for patients with chronic lymphoma and chronic leukemia. The results to date have been very encouraging.

— Joanna Zhao, Professor at Five Branches Institute, College of Traditional Medicine and Clinical Director at the Santa Cruz TCM Clinic

Brian Kie Weissbuch, L.Ac.

American Ginseng (radix Panax quinquefolium) is a superior tonic restorative when used appropriately. In determining suitability for a particular patient, first determine if heart, lung, and kidney heat and dryness patterns are due to an excess or deficiency condition. This is particularly important for treatment of heart disharmonies. Symptoms of heart palpitations, dizziness, insomnia, dream disturbed sleep, anxiety, irritability, red tongue, night sweats, and low fever may be associated with heart channel deficiency, excess, or both. The definitive method for determination is pulse diagnosis. A fine, small, slightly rapid pulse in the heart position is indicative of heart yin deficiency, and suggests that American ginseng may be very beneficial in restoring physical and emotional balance. Conversely, patients manifesting a deep, full and bounding pulse in the heart position or with heart Qi dominating the entire pulse, will have an adverse response to P. quinquefolium. This contraindication corresponds to Dr. Shen's conformation of "Heart Dominant."

Quality is a major concern with American Ginseng. Most of the commercial herb is "woods-grown," and sprayed frequently with several toxic agrichemicals. Ginseng farmers seeking maximum yield per acre create a product with high levels of residue. Be certain the product you are using is certified organically grown. This will increase your expense substantially, but you will have an immune tonic without immunosuppressive carcinogens negating the benefits of the herb.

—Brian Kie Weissbuch, KW Health Associates and KW Botanicals

Appendix B:
RECIPES

GINSENG VITALITY SOUP

Used together, the herbs in this recipe replenish the body's vital substances: the Qi, the Blood, and the Essence. It is appropriate at any time of the year and is especially beneficial when eaten at the beginning of every season to maintain physical strength and immunity. It is also an excellent dietary remedy to speed convalescence from colds, flu, and other debilitated conditions.

INGREDIENTS:
1 oz sliced white Chinese ginseng root (cool weather)
1 oz sliced American ginseng root (warm weather)
1 oz sliced astragalus root   1 oz sliced dioscorea rhizome
12 Chinese black dates   1 medium finger of fresh ginger root

1 medium turnip (cool weather)   1 medium daikon radish (warm weather)
2 medium carrots   3 dried or fresh shiitake mushrooms
1/2 cup fresh coriander, parsley, or watercress

8 cups vegetable or chicken stock   1 tbsp sesame oil
1/2 tsp sea salt or 1 tbsp soy sauce   1/4 cup rice wine (cool weather) (optional)
1/4 cup rice vinegar (warm weather) (optional)

PREPARATION:
Bring the soup stock to a boil in a pyrex, corning ware, or stainless steel pot, and turn down the heat to a low simmer. Add the ginseng, astragalus, dioscorea, and ginger. Cover the pot and cook for 1 hour.

While the herbs are cooking, wash the dates in cold water, then blanch in boiling water for 1 minute to soften them. After 1 minute place them immediately in cold water, remove the pits and put aside. If using dried shiitake mushrooms, first wash in cold water then place in a bowl of hot water to soak. When mushrooms have swelled up, remove from soak water, cut off stems, slice into thin strips and put aside. If using fresh shiitake mushrooms, wash in cold water, cut off stems, slice into thin strips and put aside. Peel and slice or dice the turnip or daikon and carrots and put aside. Wash greens in cold water, chop coarsely, and put aside.

After the herbs have finished cooking, strain the liquor into another pot and discard the herbs. Heat the herb stock to a simmer and add the turnip or daikon, carrots, mushrooms, and dates. Add salt or soy sauce and sesame oil. Cover the pot and simmer for about 20 minutes or until the vegetables are tender. Add rice or rice vinegar if desired, turn off heat, cover pot and steep for five more minutes. Remove from stove and ladle into small or large bowls. Finally, sprinkle 1 tsp of the chopped parsley, coriander, or watercress on top of each bowl and serve.

from Harriet Beinfield, co-author *Between Heaven and Earth: A Guide to Chinese Medicine.*
© copyright 1996 Efrem Korngold and Harriet Beinfield

Ginseng Congee

1 ounce dried ginseng
1/2 cup rice
6 cups water, vegetable, or chicken broth
1/2 tsp salt

Tie ginseng (and other herbs, such as codonopsis or astragalus, if desired) in cheesecloth. Place rice, water, and herbs in a heavy pot or crock pot. Simmer 2-4 hours. Remove herb sack. Garnish with scallions and soy sauce. Serve.

Makes 6 cups.

from Sharon Malley, natural foods and herbal cooking instructor

Ginseng Chicken Soup

I truly believe, as do the Chinese, that Ginseng has life-enhancing powers. The technique of cooking this soup in a heatproof bowl placed inside a larger cooking pot is a classic cooking technique for making the most flavorful broth.

INGREDIENTS:
8 soaked shiitake (black mushrooms) thinly sliced
2 chicken breasts, skinned   2 chicken thighs, skinned and fat cut away
4 cups freshly-made chicken stock   1 medium size reishi mushroom thinly sliced
4 ginseng roots, total weight 1 oz (use white American ginseng in the summer, because of its cooling effect; in the winter use Kirin cured Red Chinese ginseng for its warming effect)

PREPARATION:
Trim fat from chicken. Blanch chicken in boiling water for 1 minute: drain. Transfer all ingredients to an earthenware pot with a top. Cover with lid and set aside.

COOKING:
Pour 2 cups water into a deep 8 quart stockpot. Place the covered earthenware pot into the deep 8 quart stockpot. Add more water until it reaches halfway up the side of the inner outside of earthenware pot. Cover the stockpot with lid and bring water to a boil. Cook over medium-high heat for 4 hours. Add additional water to stockpot as needed. *Note: To provide the maximum heat needed to keep the soup simmering, keep the water in the stockpot at a vigorous boil. Also keep another large pot of water boiling to add to your 8 quart stockpot as needed in order to maintain maximum heat.*
Makes 4 servings.

From Rev. Nam Singh O.M.D., chef specialist in cooking with Chinese herbs

APPENDIX C: RESOURCES
SOURCES FOR GINSENG AND RELATED HERBS

Blessed Herbs
109 Barrie Plains Rd.
Oakham, MA 01068
800 489-4372
fresh and dry ginseng roots

Companion Plants
7247 N. Coolville Ridge Rd.
Athens, OH 45701
614 592-4643
live ginseng plants

Dabney Herbs
PO Box 22061
Lewisville, KY 40252
502 893-5198
dry ginseng roots

Gardens of the Blue Ridge
PO Box 10
US 221 North
Pineola, NC 28662
704 733-2417
ginseng seeds and live plants

Ginsana (G115)
*standardized ginseng extract in capsules
available at drugstores and health food stores*

Ginseng America Incorporated
PO Box 246
Roxbury, NY 12474
800 917-7719
607 326-3123
plants, crowns, seeds, bulk roots, products

Ginseng Board of Wisconsin
16 H Menard Plaza
Wausau, WI 54401
715 845-7300
*facilitators of buying and selling Wisconsin
ginseng*

Great China Herb Company
857 Washington St.
San Francisco, CA 94108
415 982-2195
Chinese herbs, ginseng in bulk

Herb Pharm
Box 116
Williams, OR 97544
800 348-4372
*woods-grown, Korean, and Siberian ginseng
tinctures*

Herbs Etc.
1345 Cerrillos Rd.
Santa Fe, NM 87505
800 634-3727
*Chinese Kirin, Korean white, wild
American, woods-grown, mixed ginsengs,
and Siberian ginseng tinctures*

Mayway U.S.A.
1338 Cypress St.
Oakland, CA 94607
510 208-3113
*Chinese herbs, ginseng roots and powders,
extracts*

New York Ginseng Association
PO Box 127
Roxbury, NY 12474
607 326-3005
*educational resource; organization for
growers and other people interested in
ginseng*

Rainbow Light
207 McPherson
Santa Cruz, CA 95060
800 635-1233
800 227-0555 (in California)
*woods-grown ginseng, mixed ginsengs,
and Siberian ginseng tinctures*

Recommended Reading

Ginseng Cultivation
Ginseng, How to Find, Grow, and Use America's Forest Gold by K.D. Pritts. Stackpole Books. 1995.

Inspirational Tapes and Books
The Present Moment by Thich Nhat Hanh. (audiotape)
The Inner Art of Meditation by Jack Kornfield. (audiotape)
The Art of Good Living by Svevo Brooks. (book)
Creating Health by Deepak Chopra. (book)
Love, Medicine, and Miracles by Bernie Siegel. (book)
Yoga for Beginners from *Yoga Journal*. (videotape)

General Reading on Chinese Medicine
Between Heaven and Earth, A Guide to Chinese Medicine by Harriet Beinfield and Efrem Korngold.
Chinese Herbal Medicine by Daniel Reid.
Chinese Materia Medica by Bensky and Gamble.
Glossary of Chinese Medical Terms by N. Wiseman.
Herbal Emissaries by S. Foster and Y. Chongxi.
Planetary Herbology by Michael Tierra.
The Illustrated Chinese Materia Medica by K.Y. Yen.
The Web That Has No Weaver by Ted Kaptchuk.

Appendix D:
CHEMICAL CONSTITUENTS OF GINSENG

Although ginseng (*P. ginseng*) has been used clinically for thousands of years, it was only in the 1950s that scientists began to successfully characterize the biologically active ingredients that make it work. They are called saponins, 4-ring steroid-like chemicals with attached sugar molecules that make a foam when shaken in water. In the early 1960s, Russian and Japanese researchers identified specific saponins unique to ginseng, dubbed "ginsenosides" or "panaxosides," after "panax."

TABLE 6. STEROID SAPONIN CONTENT OF GINSENG SPECIES

Species	Total Saponins
Panax ginseng	1.6-4.4%
Panax quinquefolius	4.3-4.9%
Panax notoginseng	8.2-20.6%
Panax japonica var. *major*	ca. 9.34%

[Taken from Huang, 1993; Wang et al, 1982]

To be sure, ginseng contains many other compounds as well, depending on the time of year it is harvested, the soil in which it is growing, and other factors. By weight, the major constituents are included in the following table:

TABLE 7: MAJOR CONSTITUENTS OF GINSENG

Fiber 59,000-245,000 ppm
  Soluble: pectin, starch (80,000-320,000 ppm), polysaccharides
  Insoluble: cellulose
  Heteropolysaccharides: panaxans A, B, C. D, E; ginsenan S-IA and ginsenan S-IIA
    (stimulates phagocytosis in the reticuloendothelial system) (Tomoda, 1993)

Simple sugars (about 5%)
  Fructose 4,000 ppm
  Rhamnose (1,900 ppm)
  Sucrose (85,000 ppm)
  D-glucose 5-10,000 ppm

Lipids (1.5-1.9%) (Choi et al, 1985)

Vitamins
  Niacin 60 ppm

(Table 7: Con't)

Minerals (Cho & Lee, 1983; Wei & An, 1983)
 Cadmium 0.4 ppm
 Calcium 2,340-11,000 (167.3-6,904.8) ppm
 Copper 3.7-24.6 ppm
 Germanium (amount not available)
 Iron 49-407 (74.3-518.9) ppm
 Lead 2 ppm
 Magnesium 980 (749.9-8,928.9) ppm
 Manganese 55-156 (12.9-4119.8) ppm
 Molybdenum 0.1 ppm
 Phosphorus 2,700-5,200 ppm
 Potassium 6,600 (2,622.2-17,672.0) ppm
 Sodium 35.3-6,204.3 ppm
 Zinc 15.2-75.2 ppm

Proteins
 Peptide glycans (panaxans)
 Polypeptides RGPI, RGPII (Wu et al, 1991)
 Amino Acids: arginine (11,530 ppm), glutamic acid (4,450 ppm), glycine (1,540 ppm),
  serine (1,240 ppm), lysine (2,000 ppm), etc., adenosine, pyro-glutamic acid.

Phenolic compounds
 Maltol (Huang, 1993) major phenolic compound, stable antioxidant (Kim et al, 1984)–
  same as p-hydroxycinnamic acid (Han et al, 1981)
 Salicylic acid (0.0076%) (*Huang, 1993*)
 Vanillic acid (0.0033%) (Han et al, 1981)

Terpenes
 Acetylenic compounds (panaxynol, panaxydol, panaxytriol): cytotoxic
  (Matsunaga et al, 1995)
 Essential oil (0.05%) (consisting of eremophilene, ⟨β-gurjunene, caryophyllene,
  ε-muurolene, γ-patchoulene, β-eudesmol, β-farnesene, β-bisabolene,
  aromadendrene, and other compounds)

Triterpenes
 Saponin glycosides (ginsenosides, 7,500-10,000 ppm)*
 Steroid alcohols
 Beta-sitosterol (5,000 ppm)
 Stigmasterol

Miscellaneous compounds
pyruvic acid, choline, and a number of others (see Duke, 1989)

*For more information on the chemistry of the genus Panax, see Shoji (1985), Shibata et al
(1985), Duke (1989), Chong & Oberholzer (1988), and Tang & Eisenbrand (1992).*

Of all the many known compounds in ginseng, it is the ginsenosides that make it unique. Ginsenosides are common to all the true ginsengs—whether *Panax ginseng* or *Panax quinquefolius* or *Panax notoginseng* in the amount of from 1-7%—and they do not exist in other plants. However, there are up to eleven major ginsenosides and approximately nineteen others occurring in minor amounts in all *Panax* species, and their actual individual levels tend to differ for each species, or with the type of processing used, and other growing conditions (Chuang et al, 1995). Red ginseng, for example, contains the ginsenosides that are in white ginseng, plus a few others that are apparently created during the steam-heat process (Shibata et al, 1985).

A good ginseng product should contain a minimum amount of ginsenosides. For instance, ginseng is currently included in the French Pharmacopeia, which calls for at least 2% ginsenosides to be present. A number of tests, including thin-layer chromatography (TLC), high-performance liquid chromatography (HPLC), and colorimetric analysis are used to determine the identity and quality of ginseng products in France, Germany, and other countries. Unfortunately, products for sale in countries around the world are not all carefully tested, and many inferior products are sold. Researchers from Taiwan tested thirty-seven commercial samples of ginseng from different parts of Asia and found that they varied widely in ginsenoside content and identity (Chuang et al, 1995). We have included some helpful guidelines for the selection of the best ginseng products under the "Ginseng Supplements" section.

It is interesting to note the total content of ginsenosides in the major commercial species of *Panax*, which is noted in the table below. Although *P. notoginseng* has up to five times more ginsenosides than *P. ginseng*, it is used primarily as an anti-inflammatory and pain-relieving herb and also to regulate bleeding, as discussed elsewhere in this book. There may be other compounds present in *P. notoginseng*, or perhaps the proportions of individual ginsenosides are different enough to alter its activity.

Although the root is the preferred medicinal part of ginseng, the leaf has up to twice the ginsenoside content (Samukawa et al, 1995). The leaf is not used medically but is preferred as a restorative tea. Ginseng leaf tea is much less expensive than the root, so it is no doubt a good buy, and the taste is rather pleasant.

PHARMACOLOGY & ACTIONS—
EFFECTS OF GINSENG

The pharmacology, or the mechanisms by which the individual constituents and whole plant extracts affect body processes, of ginseng is very complex. In this section, we provide an overview of many of these effects. Literally hundreds of laboratory tests have been performed with animals, which have shown various ginseng extracts to have antifatigue, central nervous system stimulating, and hypotensive effects. They were also able to stimulate respiration, provide protection against stress ulcer, accelerate glycolysis, cholesterol synthesis (serum and liver), nuclear RNA synthesis, and serum protein synthesis, lower blood sugar by potentiating the action of insulin, raise the red blood cell and hemoglobin count, have a tranquilizing action, induce a serotonic-like effect, have an anti-inflammatory and antipyretic action as well as an antihistamine-like and antipsychotic activity (Shibata et al, 1985). The ginseng extracts were administered mostly by injection, but also orally in various dosages.

Scientists are concerned not only with what effects drugs and herbal extracts have on the body, but how they produce these effects. What are the physiological pathways by which individual constituents work their magic? These are among the most difficult questions to answer, because all body processes are fundamentally intertwined so that by affecting one enzyme, for instance, a host of other reactions and processes might be affected. For ginseng and especially the ginsenosides, a number of biochemical effects have been observed and from these observations, several major mechanisms are proposed to explain the activity of ginseng. These include:

➤ Stimulation of RNA and DNA synthesis in blood, liver, and other cells
➤ Increase of the size of mitochondria, the organelle that provides energy, the "power pack" of the cell
➤ Stimulation of ACTH production from the pituitary gland; ACTH is a hormone that stimulates further production of hormones from the adrenal glands
➤ Stimulation of nerve growth-factor (NGF)
➤ Potent inhibition of Calcium channels in sensory neurons, reducing secretion of neurotransmitters and mimicking the action of opioids without activating opioid receptors; present in very small amounts in most ginseng (Nah et al, 1995)

➤ Enhancement of macrophage activity
➤ Interactions with central cholinergic (Benishin et al, 1991) and
   dopaminergic mechanisms (Watanabe et al, 1991)
➤ Enhancement of neurotransmitter activity (Quiroga, 1982)
[From Shibata et al (1985), except where noted]

As the most widely studied of ginseng's constituents, the
ginsenosides have individual names. The two main ones are Rb1 and
Rg1. In animals, they have opposite effects. Rb1 tends to suppress the
central nervous system, while Rg1 is a stimulant (Chong and
Oberholzer, 1988). Rb1 is also tranquilizing and blood-pressure-
lowering (hypotensive), while Rg1 is also blood-pressure-raising
(hypertensive) and has an anti-fatigue effect. The following table
reviews many of the ginsenosides identified from *P. ginseng*, their
percentages, and major pharmacological effects.

TABLE 8: THE MAJOR GINSENOSIDES AND THEIR PHARMACOLOGY

Ginsenoside	Amount	Major Effects, Notes
Ro	0.2-0.4%	—
Ra1	0.02%	—
Ra2	0.03%	—
Ra3	trace	—
Rb	x	stimulation of cholesterol synthesis
Rb1	0.37-0.5%	Stimulant action on protein and RNA synthesis in animal serum and liver; hypotensive, anticonvulsant, analgesic; antiulcer (induced by stress), nerve regeneration-inducing effect (nerve growth factor induction)
Rb3	trace	—
Rc	0.13-0.3%	stimulation of serum protein synthesis: potent stimulation of adrenal steroid output
Rd	0.15%	stimulation of adrenal intracellular cAMP
Re	0.15-0.20%	
Rf	0.05%	—
Rg	0.05%	
Rg1	0.2%	stimulant action on DNA, protein and lipid synthesis in animal bone marrow cells, CNS-stimulating, hypertensive, antifatigue, increase of initial learning response
Rg2	trace	characteristic in red ginseng
Rg3	trace	characteristic in red ginseng
Rh1	trace	hepatoprotective, antitumor activity, hepatoprotective; characteristic in red ginseng
Rs1	trace	—
Rs2	trace	—
mRb1	—	acidic malonates of the dammarane saponins (malonylginsenosides)
mRb2	—	acidic malonates of the dammarane saponins (malonylginsenosides)
mRc	—	acidic malonates of the dammarane saponins (malonylginsenosides)

Note: Ginsenosides Rg2, Rg3, Rh1, and Rh2 are known to be breakdown products of ginsenosides Rb1, Rb2, Rc, and Rd during the steaming of white ginseng and the creation of red ginseng. They do not occur in white ginseng in significant amounts, but do occur in red ginseng in small amounts. These compounds may also be created during the process of making tea with white ginseng (Shoji, 1985).

**Data summarized from Shibata et al (1985), Shoji (1985), Huang (1993), Thompson (1991), Chang & But (1986), Tang & Eisenbrand (1992), Chuang et al (1995).

Table 9 reviews the major pharmacological effects of whole ginseng extracts or the total ginsenosides. The total saponins and whole ginseng extracts are mostly administered to mice and rats by injection (i.p. or i.v.).

TABLE 9: MAJOR PHARMACOLOGICAL EFFECTS OF WHOLE GINSENG EXTRACTS

EFFECTS ON PERFORMANCE, MENTAL AND PHYSICAL WELL-BEING
- General stimulation of pituitary-adrenal axis
- Anti-fatigue effect
- Slight central-nervous system (CNS) stimulation
- Anti-anxiety effect for white and red ginseng (50 mg/kg x 5 days) administered to rats (Bhattacharya & Mitra, 1991)
- Improvement in memory and learning at low dose (Petkov & Mosharrof, 1987)
- Locomotor activity increased at high dose (Petkov & Mosharrof, 1987)
- Adrenal stimulation
- Short-term doses of large amounts of ginseng stimulate thyroid function, long-term use depresses
- Increased production of ACTH by pituitary (plasma ACTH was increased by oral feeding of total ginsenosides) with corresponding fall in corticosterone
- Pain-relieving activity
- Red blood cell production from bone marrow, increased red blood cell incorporation of iron
- CNS-depressant activity
- Smooth muscle-relaxing activity

PROTECTIVE EFFECTS
- General adrenal-protective effect
- Antioxidant effect (maltol; salicylic, vanillic acids)
- Increased blood clearance of alcohol, faster recovery from alcohol intoxication
- Hepatoprotective effect after liver damage by chronic alcohol exposure
- Reduction in blood glucose (panaxans)
- Increased blood insulin levels, reduced blood sugar
- Lipolysis inhibition and lipogenesis stimulation from pyro-glutamic acid with insulin-like activity (Takaku et al, 1990)
- Reduction of triglycerides, cholesterol levels in blood
- Reduction of, or increase in blood pressure, depending on dose and method of administration. Ginseng water extract enhanced the growth of beneficial human gut microflora, including *Bifidobacteria* spp. (Ahn, et al, 1990)
- Protective effect against exposure to radiation
- Anti-inflammatory effect externally when applied to burns
- Heart muscle-protective effect in mice, dogs, and rabbits
- Antiarrhythmic effects in mice
- Hepatoprotective effect
- Antihistamine-like activity (another test was negative)
- Protective effect on aorta endothelium subsequent to high lipid diet (protects against atherosclerosis formation, HDL levels were elevated)

HORMONAL EFFECTS AND EFFECTS ON SEXUAL SYSTEM
- Hormone-like effects (oral dose)
- Blood testosterone levels were significantly increased, and prostate size was reduced after 30 days of an addition of 5% ginseng to the diet of rats (Fahim et al, 1982)
- Increased sperm counts in rabbit testes (Chang & But, 1986)
- Estrogen-like effect directly on vaginal epithelium with no increase in serum estrogen
- Strong estrogenic effect in rats (Chang & But, 1986)
- No detectable estrogenic effects in female juvenile rats (Büchi & Jenny, 1984)

IMMUNE SYSTEM EFFECTS
- •Increases phagocytic activity of the reticuloendothelial system
- •Increase of antibody response (IgG, IgM) and natural killer cell activity
- •Increased protection against viral infection when used with chemotherapy
- •Protects against white blood cell count reduction during bacterial infection

*Above data summarized from Chong & Oberholzer (1988), Shibata et al (1985), Huang (1993), Thompson (1987), Chang & But (1986), Tang & Eisenbrand (1992).
**See Petkov & Mosharrof (1987) for a summary of Bulgarian research on the effects of a standardized ginseng extract (G115) and other ginseng extracts on memory and learning in animals and humans.

Absorption of Ginsenosides

Some animal studies report that many of the ginsenosides are absorbed rapidly from the upper digestive tract. The total amount varies, depending on a number of factors, such as stomach acidity and the specific compound. For instance, from 2-30% of Rg1 was absorbed within 30 minutes to an hour (Odani et al, 1983a; Strombom et al, 1985), while very little of Rb1 was absorbed (Odani et al, 1983b). The dose seems to markedly affect the absorption of the compounds. Doses higher than the traditional recommended dose of 3-9 grams (or an equivalent amount of extract) result in less efficient absorption (Han et al, 1986). Other studies show that after 20-26 hours, from 2-45% of the total amount is excreted (Han et al, 1986). In most animal studies, maximum blood levels are reached within 30 minutes, and tissue levels are highest in about 1.5 hours. Absorption may differ some in humans, but probably not significantly. Tinctures (alcoholic extracts) of ginseng and other types of extracts (teas, powdered extracts) are more rapidly absorbed than whole roots, because the active constituents are freed from the cell wall structures, rendering them more available.

Ginsenosides are excreted from the urine mostly in unmetabolized form (Huang, 1993).

There are so many effects to point to in the countless animal studies performed on ginseng and its constituent compounds, that one can't help but wonder, what is the bottom line? Modern medicine often scoffs at so many contradictory and seemingly diverse effects, but again, with adaptogens and herbal medicines working slowly to bring about a balance in the physiological functions of the body, these can be considered reasonable results. Because many of the physiological effects are subtle, it is necessary to look closely at the traditional uses of the ginsengs to determine the optimum way in which to utilize them. However, the chemistry and pharmacology is of interest, and as it continues to advance, the results will have a major impact on how we look at this whole group of medicinal plants. For instance, animal studies show that the individual ginsenosides Rb-1 and Rd can potentiate nerve growth factor (NGF), which can have the ability to help nerves regenerate to a certain degree. When we consider that American ginseng has about three times the amount of both of these constituents in their roots than white or red Asian ginseng (Shibata et al, 1985), perhaps one might choose the former when using ginseng with someone who has nerve weakness or degeneration. Whether this will work in actual practice has yet to be proven, but it points out that new information on medicinal plants via their chemistry and pharmacology may prove to be a valuable contribution to our knowledge on their effective uses.

Like the individual ginsenosides, ginseng itself has been reported to have contradictory effects. For instance, ginseng or its ginsenosides have been reported to stimulate and depress the central nervous system, as we've mentioned, but also to raise blood pressure in some cases, to lower it in others. It can stimulate, or tranquilize. It can have histaminic or anti-histamine effects. It has been reported to raise cholesterol and to lower it, to raise and lower blood sugar levels, to increase and decrease heart rate (Duke, 1989). Although these seemingly conflicting effects make sense in the light of its regulating or "amphoteric" effects, it is no wonder many scientists consider ginseng to be a medical enigma! Western drugs, by contrast, generally have only one effect. If you take a medication to lower blood pressure, in the vast majority of cases it does just that; it can also have other negative side effects as well, but that's another story.

Ginseng also seems to act differently in different people, but that's the way a drug that restores homeostasis, or balance, *should* work. As one author writing on ginseng put it:

The Oriental herbalist may use the appropriate ginseng species or type as a tea to normalize a person who is diagnosed as being excessively Yin or Yang. This philosophy is an interesting working hypothesis as ginseng is known to both stimulate or sedate, and to be either hypertensive or hypotensive (Staba and Chen, 1979).

There are two mechanisms by which ginseng can have these different effects. One is the different "energies" of the various types of ginsengs. We've noted that American ginseng is thought to be more cooling and Yin-promoting compared with Chinese or Korean ginseng, and that red ginseng's ginsenosides undergo changes that make them hotter and more "yang."

Studies confirm that American ginseng tends to have relatively more of the relaxing blood-pressure-lowering Rb1, while Korean *Panax ginseng* has more of the stimulating Rg1 (Fulder, 1993). Thus, each ginseng would have a different biological effect. If you were old and yang-deficient or suffering from an illness that made you very weak and deficient, Chinese or Korean ginseng might be appropriate. If you

INCREASED PRODUCTION OF ACTH – A MAJOR EFFECT OF GINSENG?

Ginseng appears to help tone the hormone-regulating and coordinating system in the body, the hypothalamic-pituitary-adrenal axis. It stimulates this system, which in turn tells the various glands in the body to secrete hormones, which help regulate many body functions. For instance, the concentrations of various hormones in the blood of eight volunteers (5 were healthy and 3 diabetic) were studied after a single oral dose of 4.5 to 6.0 grams of red ginseng powder. Plasma cortisol was increased in the normal volunteers and decreased in the diabetics. The hormone ACTH was increased in both groups, but blood adrenaline levels were increased or decreased, depending on the patient. This may indicate an adrenal-regulating effect. If a person is generally aroused (high sympathetic nervous system tone), ginseng can relax, and if the sympathetic tone is low, it can bring it up to normal levels.

Stephen Fulder, a ginseng researcher of note and author of the influential *Tao of Medicine* (1980), has theorized that ginseng saponins stimulate the hypothalamic-pituitary axis to secrete ACTH, which in turn has a variety of effects in the body. ACTH is known to bind directly to brain cells and affect behavior, as well as "improve motivation, performance and arousal. It can also produce a temporary feeling of vitality and well-being which is greater in debilitated and fatigued patients" (Fulder, 1981). He argues that like ACTH, the ginsenosides are known to affect the vigilance systems but not random locomotion (D'Angelo et al, 1986). Fulder also connects the traditional use of ginseng with the hormone-regulating effect of ginseng. In TCM, ginseng is recommended for certain individuals at specific times of the year. Perhaps pharmacology can have a hand at clarifying this unexplainable (at least to the western scientist) phenomenon, for science has shown that the hypothalamus adjusts its hormone levels according to the seasons (Fulder, 1981).

were under 40 or 50 and over-stressed, overstimulated, and on the road to burnout, American ginseng might have a better energy for you.

The second way that ginseng has different effects on different people, however, is that it helps maintain homeostasis, that is, balance. Our bodies have many systems that are designed to keep certain biological parameters within proper limits. For example, our blood optimally contains about 1% calcium; if it falls below 1%, our bodies will pull calcium from the bones to maintain that percentage. Probably the best-known homeostatic system is temperature. Each of us has a normal body temperature; it's not always 98.6, but it's close to that. When we get hot, we perspire; when we get cold, we shiver. Each acts to keep our internal body temperature the same.

Blood pressure, blood sugar, and many other aspects of the human body are kept under homeostatic control under normal circumstances. Many of these regulatory systems are controlled by hormones. When we are under chronic stress, however, the "stress hormones", or corticosteroids, can become elevated and interfere with homeostasis. We can literally become "hot under the collar" from stress.

Although the focus of the pharmacological research on ginseng is on the ginsenosides, a number of other proven active compounds can be found in the plant. Beta-sitosterol (5,000 ppm), for instance, is a plant steroid alcohol (from a class of plant compounds called "phytosterols") that helps lower blood cholesterol levels and has anti-tumor effects. Ginseng also has antioxidants such as selenium, vitamin C, and maltol. Compounds such as these, though, tend to be common in many plants and are not considered as interesting by scientists who often seek to find patentable and marketable drugs.

Herbalists often feel that the activity and healing energy of any medicinal plant are greater than the sum of its individual constituents, and that laboratory research can only take us so far in the understanding of its true nature and its healing relationship with us.

Bibliography

Ahn, Y-J. et al. 1981. Effect of soil fumigation treatment on the growth and the chemical composition of Korean ginseng, Panax ginseng C.A. Meyer. *Hanguk Sikmul Poha Hakhoe Chi.* 20: 31-36.

Ahn, Y-J, et al. 1990. Selective growth responses of human Intestinal bacteria to Araliaceae extracts. *Microbial Ecology in Health and Disease* 3: 223-30.

Anderson et al. 1993. The ecology and biology of Panax quinquefolium L. (Araliaceae) in Illinois. *American Midland Naturalist* 129: 357-73.

Antoniak, M. 1994. New awareness for ancient Chinese herbs. *Vitamin Retailer* (April).

Awang, D.V.C. 1991. Maternal Use of Ginseng and Neonatal Androgenization. *JAMA.* 266: 363.

Bae, H. 1978. *Korean Ginseng*, 2nd ed. Republic of Korea: Korean Ginseng Research Institute.

Barenboim, D. 1986. *Eleutherococcus senticosus.* Moscow: Medexport.

Beinfield, H. and E. Korngold. 1991. *Between Heaven and Earth.* New York: Ballantine.

Benishin, C.G. et al. 1991. Effects of ginsenoside Rb-1 on central cholinergic metabolism. *Pharmacology.* 42: 223-29.

Bensky, D. & A. Gamble. 1986. *Chinese Materia Medica.* Seattle: Eastland Press.

Bergner, P. 1992. Using Three Common Herbs Wisely. *Natural Health.* Jan-Feb, 22: 33.

Bespalov, V.G. et al. 1993. Inhibition of mammary gland carcinogenesis using a tincture from biomass of ginseng tissue culture. *Biulleten Eksperimentalnoi Biologii i Meditsiny.* 115: 59-61.

Bhattacharya, S.K. and S.K. Mitra. 1991. Anxiolytic activity of Panax ginseng roots: an experimental study. *Journal of Ethnopharmacology.* 34: 87-92.

Bigelow, J. 1817. *American Medical Botany.* Boston: Cummings and Hilliard.

Blumenthal, M. 1996. *Commission E Herbal Monographs.* Austin: American Botanical Council. (In press).

Blumenthal, M. 1991. "Debunking the Ginseng Abuse Syndrome," *Whole Foods.* March.

Bradley, P.R. 1992. *British Herbal Compendium.* Dorset: British Herbal Medicine Association.

Bretschneider, E. 1895. *Botanicon Sinicum*, Part III. Hongkong: Kelly & Walsh, Ltd.

Büchi, K. & E. Jenny. 1984. On the interference of the standardized Ginseng Extract G115 and pure ginsenosides with agonists of the progesterone receptor of human myometrium. January 18 (unpublished).

Buchwald, D. et al. 1995. Chronic fatigue and the chronic fatigue syndrome; prevalence in a Pacific Northwest healthcare system *Annals of Internal Medicine* 123: 81-88.

Business Brief. 1995. Farming unit posts record harvest of ginseng root. (farming subsidiary of Chai-Na-Ta Corp.) *Wall Street Journal* (Thu, Nov 30):B12(W), col 2.

Carpenter, S. and G. Cottam. 1983. Growth and reproduction of American ginseng (Panax quinquefolius) in Wisconsin. *Can. J . Bot.* 60: 2692-96.

Carr, C.J. & E. Jokl. 1986. *Enhancers of Performance and Endurance.* Hillsdale, NJ: Lawrernce Eribaum Associates.

Cha, R.J. and Q.S. Chang. 1994. Non-surgical treatment of small cell lung cancer with chemo-radio-immunotherapy and traditional Chinese medicine. *Chung Hua Nei Ko Tsa Chih.* 33: 462-466.

Chang, H.-M. & P.P.-H. But. 1986. *Pharmacology and Applications of Chinese Materia Medica.* Philadelphia: World Scientific.

Chen, Y. and Y. Gao. 1994. Research on the mechanism of blood-tonifying effect of Danggui Buxue decoction. *Zhongguo Zhongyao Zazhi.* 19: 43-45, 63.

Chin, R. K. H. 1991. Ginseng and Common Pregnancy Disorders. Chinese Department of Obstretrics and Gynecology, Caritas Medical Centre, 111 Wing Hong Street, Lowloon, Hong Kong.

Cho, Y.H. and J.S. Lee. 1983. Behavior of some metallic ions in the process of ginseng extracts preparations. *Hanguk Sikp'um Kwahakhoe Chi* 15:133-35.Choi, C.W. et al. 1984. Effect of ginseng on the hepatic alcohol-metabolizing enzyme system activity in chronic alcohol-treated mouse. *Taehan Yakrihak Chapchi.* 20: 13-21.

Choi, J. H. et al. 1983. Study on stability of red and white ginseng by the number of storage years. *Hanguk Yongyang Siklyong Hakhoechi.*

Choi, J. H. et al. 1984. Studies on stability for the quality of ginseng products. Improvement of physical properties of spray dried red ginseng extract powder after moisture sorption. *Han'guk Yangyang Siklyang Hakhoechi.* 13: 251-58.

Choi, K. et al. 1983. Effect of solvents on the yield, brown color intensity, UV absorbance, reducing and antioxidant activities of extracts from white and red ginseng. *Hanguk Nonghwa Hakhoe Chi.* 26: 8-18.

Choi, K. et al. 1985. Studies on the lipid components of fresh ginseng, red ginseng and white ginseng. *Saengyak Hakhoechi.* 16: 141-50.

Chong, S.K.F and V.G. Oberholzer. 1988. Ginseng—is there a use in clinical medicine? *Postgraduate Medical Journal.* 64: 841-46.

Choy, Y.M. et al. 1994. Immunopharmacological studies of low molecular weight polysaccharide from Angelica sinensis. *American Journal Of Chinese Medicine.* 22: 137-45.

Chuang, W.-C. et al. 1995. A Comparative study on commercial samples of Ginseng Radix. *Planta Med.* 61: 459-65.

Coxe, J.R. 1830. *The American Dispensatory.* Philadelphia: Carey & Lea.

D'Angelo, L. et al. 1986. A double-blind, placebo-controlled clinical study on the effect of a standardized ginseng extract on psychomotor performance in healthy volunteers. *J. Ethnopharmacol.* 16: 15-22. *Deutsches Arzneibuch.* 10.Ausgabe. 1991. Stuttgart: Deutscher Apotheker Verlag (DAB10).

Deveny, K. 1992. Garlic pills are potent drugstore sellers. *Wall Street Journal* (Thu, Oct 1):B1(W), B1(E), col 4, 31 col in.

Ding, D.Z. 1995. Effects of red ginseng on the congestive heart failure and its mechanism. *Chung Kuo Chung Hsi I Chieh Ho Tsa Chih.* 15: 325-27.

Dörling, E. et al. 1980. Haben Ginsenoside Einfluss auf das Leistungsvermögen? Ergebnisse einer Doppelblindstudie. *Notabene Medici* 10: 241-46.

Dubos, R. 1965. *Man Adapting.* New Haven: Yale University Press.

Duke, J.A. 1989. *Ginseng: A Concise Handbook.* Algonac, MI: Reference Publications, Inc.

Editors of Consumer Reports. 1995. Herbal Roulette. *Consumer Reports,* 698-705.

Elden, H.R. 1990. Ginsenosides—New Uses for an Old Root. *Drug and Cosmetic Industry.* April.

Fahim, M.S. et al. 1982. Effect of *Panax ginseng* on testosterone level and prostate in male rats. *Arch. Andrology* 8: 261-64.

Farnsworth, N.R. et al. 1985. Siberian Ginseng (*Eleutherococcus senticosus*): Current Status as an Adaptogen. In Wagner, H. and N. Farnsworth (eds.), *Economic and Medicinal Plant Research,* vol. 1. New York: Academic Press.

Felter, H.W. & J.U. Lloyd. 1898. *King's American Dispensatory*. Cincinnati: The Ohio Valley Co.

Feng, S.L. and C.S. Song. 1985. 32 cases of chronic bronchitis treated with a mixture of Codonopsis pilosula and the feces of Trogopteri. *Chung Hsi I Chieh Ho Tsa Chih*. (Feb) 5: 102-104, 68-69.

Forgo, I. 1980. Effect of a standardized ginseng extract on general health, reactive capacity and pulmonary function. *Proceedings of the 3rd International Ginseng Symposium*. Seoul: Korea Ginseng Research Institute.

Forgo, I. et al. 1981. Effect of a standardized ginseng extract on general well-being, reaction capacity, pulmonary function and gonadal hormones. *Medizinische Welt* 32: 751-56.

Forgo, I. and A.M. Kirchdorfer. 1981. On the question of influencing the performance of top sportsmen by means of biologically active substances. *Aerztliche Praxis* 33: 1784-86.

Forgo, I. 1983. Effects of drugs on physical performance and hormone system of sportsmen. *Münchener Medizinische Wochenschrift* 125: 822-24.

Forgo, I. & G. Schimert. 1985. *Notabene Mecici*. 15: 636-40.

Foster, S. and Y. Chongxi. 1992. *Herbal Emissaries*. Rochester, VT: Healing Arts Press.

Fryer, L. 1995. The Wisconsin Ginseng Project. *Acres, U.S.A.* (June), p. 8-9ff.

Fulder, S. 1981. Ginseng and the hypothalamic-pituitary control of stress. *American J. of Chinese Med.* 9: 112-18.

Fulder, S. 1993. *The Book of Ginseng and other Chinese herbs for vitality*. Rochester, Vermont: Healing Arts Press; originally published in 1980 at *The Tao of Medicine*.

Gathercoal, E.N. and H.W. Youngken. 1942. *Check List of Native and Introduced Drug Plants in the United States*. Chicago: National Research Council.

Goolrick, C. 1983. Hong Kong will get its ginseng if snakes don't get the digger; Appalachian hill folk brave wilds to find root valued by culture a world away. *Wall Street Journal* (Thu, March 3):1(W), 1(E), col 4.

Griffith, R.E. 1847. *Medical Botany*. Philadelphia: Lea & Blanchard.

Hallstrom, C. et al. 1982. Effects of Ginseng on the Performance of Nurses on Night Duty. *Comparative Medicine East and West*. 6: 277-82.

Han, B.H. et al. 1986. Studies on the metabolic fates of ginsenosides. *Korean Biochem*. 19: 213-18.

Han, B.H. et al. 1983 Studies on the antioxidant components of Korean ginseng. III. Identification of phenolic acids. *Arch. Pharmacol. Res.* 4: 53058.

Hess, F.G. et al. 1983. Effects of subronic feeding of ginseng extract G115 in beagle dogs. *Food Chem. Toxicol*. 21: 95-97.

Hopkins, M.P. et al. 1988. Ginseng face cream and unexplained vaginal bleeding. *Am. J. Obstet. Gynecol*. 159: 1121-22.

Hsu, H.Y. et al. 1986. *Oriental Materia Medica: a concise guide*. Long Beach: Oriental Healing Arts.

Hu, S.Y. 1976. The Genus *Panax* (Ginseng) in Chinese Medicine. *Economic Botany* 30: 11-28.

Hu, Y. et al. 1992. Effects of artificial cultured Panax notoginseng cell on cardiovascular system. *Chung Kuo Chung Yao Tsa Chih*. (June) 17: 361-363, 384.

Huang, K.C. 1993. *The Pharmacology of Chinese Herbs*. Boca Raton, FL: CRC Press.

Ingersoll, B. 1992. Traders from Asia flock to Wisconsin, seeking their roots; they scramble to buy ginseng grown here, and why not? Ours can bolster their yin. *Wall Street Journal* (Fri, Nov 20):A1(W), A1(E), col 4.

Iwabuchi, H. et al. 1990. Studies on the sesquiterpenoids of Panax ginseng C.A. Meyer. IV. *Chemical and Pharmaceutical Bulletin.* 38: 1405-07.

Jang, J. G. et al. 1983. Study on the changes of saponin contents in relation to root age of Panax ginseng. *Han'guk Yangyang Siklyang Hakhoechi.* 12: 37-40.

Johnson, A. et al. 1980. Whole Ginseng Effects on Human Response to Demands for Performance. *Proceedings of the 3rd International Ginseng Symposium.* Korea Ginseng Research Institute.

Kaptchuk, T.J. 1983. *The web that has no weaver.* New York: Congdon & Weed, Inc.

Karikura, M. et al. 1992. Studies on absorption, distribution, excretion and metabolism of ginseng saponins. VIII isotope labeling of ginsenoside Rb2. *Chemical and Pharmaceutical Bulletin.* 38: 1405-07.

Kiesewetter, H. 1992. Hemorrheological and circulatory effects of Gincosan. *Int. J. Clin. Pharmacol. Ther. Toxicol.* 30: 97-102.

Kim, N.D. 1978. "Pharmacological Properties of Ginseng," pp. 115-158, in Bae, HW ed., *Korean Ginseng* (Korea Ginseng Research Institute); quoted in Duke, 1989, op. cit., p. 115.

Koren, G. and S. Randor et al. 1990. "Maternal ginseng use associated with neonatal androgenization," JAMA; 264: 2868.

Kwon, S.K. et al. 1986. Pesticide residues in three drugs from South Korea. *Planta Med.* 0: 155-156.

Lee, F.C. et al. 1987. Effects of Panax ginseng on blood alcohol clearance in man. *Clin. Exp. Pharmacol. Physiol.* 14: 543-46.

Lee, J.C. et al. 1983. Effect of temperature on embryo growth and germination of ginseng seed. *Proeedings of the 5th National Ginseng Conference.*

Lei, X.L. and G.C. Chiou. 1986. Cardiovascular pharmacology of Panax notoginseng (Burk) F.H. Chen and Salvia miltiorrhiza. *Am J Chin Med.* 14: 145-52.

Leung, A.Y. 1984. *Chinese Herbal Remedies.* New York: Universal Books.

Lewis, W.H. and V. Zenger. 1982. Population Dynamics of the American Ginseng, Panax quinquefolium (Araliaceae). *American Journal of Botany.* 69: 1483-90.

Li, H. et al. 1987. Effects of Codonopsis pilosula on experimental gastric ulcers in the rat. *Chung Hsi I Chieh Ho Tsa Chih* (March, 7): 163-65, 134.

Li, X. et al. 1991. Pharmacological variations of Panax ginseng C.A. Meyer during processing. *Chung Kuo Chung Yao Tsa Chih.* 16: 3-7, 62.

Liao, J.Z. et al. 1988. Pharmacologic effects of codonopsis pilosula-astragalus injection in the treatment of CHD patients. *J Tradit Chin Med.* (Mar) 8: 1-8.

Lo, A.C.T. 1995. Danggui (Angelica sinensis) affects the pharmacodynamics but not the pharmacokinetics of warfarin in rabbits. *European Journal Of Drug Metabolism And Pharmacokinetics* 20: 55-60.

Lou, B.Y. et al. 1989. Eye symptoms due to ginseng poisoning. *Yen Ko Hsueh Pao.* 5: 96-97.

Matsuda, H. et al. 1985. Pharmacological study on *Panax ginseng*: VII. Protective effect of Red Ginseng on infections. 1. On phagocytic activity of mouse RES. *Yakugaku Zasshi.* 105: 948-54.

Matsunaga, H. et al. 1995. A possible mechanism for the cytotoxicity of a polyacetylenic alcohol, panaxytriol: inhibition of mitochondrial respiration. *Cancer Chemother. Pharmacol.* 35: 29129-6.

Mei, Q.-b. et al. 1991. Advances in the pharmacological studies of radix *Angelica sinensis* (Oliv) Diels (Chinese danggui). *Chinese Medical Journal* 104: 776-81.

Ministère des Affaires Sociales et de la Solidarité. 1992. *Bulletin Officiel* No. 92/11 bis. Paris: Direction des Journaux Officiels. (English version).

Moerman, D.E. 1986. *Medicinal Plants of Native Americans*. Ann Arbor: Regents of University of Michigan.

Monoson, H. and C. Schertz. 1985. Angiosperm flora of Miller-Anderson woods nature presesrve Bureau and Putnam Counties, Illinois. *Trans Illinois State Academy of Sciences.* 78: 263-80.

Nemecek, S. 1996. Virtual Pollution. *Scientific American* 274 : 24.

Nah, Y.N. et al. 1995. A trace component of ginseng that inhibits Ca2+ channels through a pertussis toxin-sensitive G protein. *Proceedings of the National Academy of Science.* 92: 8739-43.

Noh, H. W. et al. 1983. Effect of relative humidity on the quality of white ginseng during storage. II. Changes in saponins and sugars. *Hanguk Sikp'um Kwahakhoe Chi.* 15: 32-36.

Odani, T. et al. 1983a. Studies on the absorption, distribution, excretion and metabolism of ginseng. *Chem. Pharm. Bull.* 31: 292-98.

Odani, T. et al. 1983b. The absorption, distribution, excretion and metabolism of ginseng saponins:3. The absorption, distribution and excretion of ginsenoside Rb1 in the rat. *Chem. Pharm. Bull.* (Tokyo) 31: 1059-66.

Osol, A. and G. E. Farrar. 1947. *The Dispensatory of the United States of America. The 24th Edition*. Philidelphia: J.B. Lippincott Co.

Owen, R.T. Ginseng - A Pharmacological Profile. *Drugs of Today*, 17(8): 343-51; 1981; quoted in Duke, J.A. op. cit., p. 115.

Pae, P. 1993. The gold grows wild in the hills of Loudoun. (farmers and landowners in Loudoun County, Virginia keep quiet about wild ginseng growing on their property for fear of poaching). *Washington Post* 116 (Sun, June 20): B5, col 1.

Parks, M. 1983. China: new pep from old tonics. *Los Angeles Times.* (Jan. 8). 102; 1, col 1, 47 col in.

Petkov, V.D. et al. 1987. Effects of standardized ginseng extract on learning, memory and physical capabilities. *American J. Chinese Med.* 15: 19-27.

Pieralisi, G. et al. 1991. Effects of a standardized ginseng extract combined with dimethylaminoethanol bitartrate, vitamins, minerals, and trace elements on physical performance during exercise. *Clin. Ther.* 13: 373-82.

Popov, I. Et al. 1974. Clinical Use of Ginseng Extract as Adjuvant in Revitalisation Therapies. *Proceedings of International Ginseng Symposium*. Republic of Korea: The Research Institute.

Proctor, J.T.A. and D.P. Ormrod. 1981. Sensitivity of ginseng to ozone and sulfur dioxide. *Horticulture Science.* 16: 647-48.

Quiroga, H.A. and A. Imbriano. 1979. The effect of Panax Ginseng extract on cerebrovascular deficits. *Orientación Médica.* 1208: 86-87.

Quiroga, H.A. 1982. Comparative double-blind study of the effect of Ginsana G115® and Hydergin® on cerebrovascular deficits. *Orientación Médica.* 1281: 201-02.

Reynolds, J. 1993. *Martindale, The Extra Pharmacopoeia*. London: The Pharmaceutical Press.

Revers, W.J. et al. 1976. Psychological effects of a geriatric preparation in the aged. *Zeitschrift für präklinische und klinische Geriatrie* 6: 418-30.

Rosenfeld, M.S. 1989. Evaluation of the efficacy of a standardized ginseng extract in patients with psychophysical asthenia and neurological disorders. *La Semana Médica* 173: 148-54.

Ryu, S.J. and Y.Y. Chien. 1995. Ginseng-associated cerebral arteritis. *Neurology* 45: 829-30.

Samukawa, K. et al. 1995. Simultaneous analysis of ginsenosides of various ginseng radix by HPLC. *Yakugaku Zasshi*. Journal of the Pharmaceutical Society of Japan. 115: 241-49.

Sandberg, F. 1974. Clinical effects of ginseng preparations. *Zeitschrift für präklinische Geriatrie*. 4: 264-68.

Sandberg, F. 1980. Vitality and senility—The effects of the ginsenosides on performance. *Svensk Farmaceitisk Tidskrift*. 84: 499-502.

Scaglione, F. et al. 1990. Immunomodulatory Effects of Two Extracts of *Panax* Ginseng C.A. Meyer. *Drugs Exptl. Clinical Research*. 16: 537-42.

Schmalzer, P.A. et al. 1985. Vascular flora of the Obed wild and scenic river, Tennessee [USA]. *Castanea*. 47: 261-65.

Schmidt, U.J. et al. 1978. Pharmacotherapy and so-called basic therapy in old age. *Xithe International Congress of Gerontology*, Tokyo, August 20-25.

Shi, L. et al. 1990. Effects of total saponins of Panax notoginseng on increasing PGI2 in carotid artery and decreasing TXA2 in blood platelets. *Chung Kuo Yao Li Hsueh Pao*. 11: 29-32.

Shi, M. 1995. Research on the stimulating action of Carthamus tinctorius L., Angelica sinensis (Oliv.) Diels and Leonurus sibiricus L. on uterus. *Zhongguo Zhongyao Zazhi*. 20: 173-75, 192. (through Biological Abstracts, BA98382073).

Shia, G.T.W. et al. 1982. The effects of Ginseng saponins on the growth and metabolism of human diploid fibroblasts. *Gerontology*. 28: 121-24.

Shibata, S. et al. 1985. Chemistry and Pharmacology of *Panax. Economic and Medicinal Plant Research, Volume 1*, Academic Press, 1985. p. 218. London: Academic Press.

Shoji, J. 1985. Recent Advances in the Chemical Studies on Ginseng. In Chang, H.M et al (eds.). *Advances in Chinese Medicinal Materials Research*. Philadelphia: World Scientific Publishing Co.

Siegel, R.K. 1979, Ginseng Abuse Syndrome. *JAMA*. 241: 15; 1614-15.

Smith, B.S. 1810. *Collections for an Essay Towards a Materia Medica of the United States*. Philadelphia: Edward Earle and Co.

Smith, F.P. and G.A. Stuart. 1973. *Chinese Medicinal Herbs*. San Francisco: Georgetown Press, 1973. (Partial translation of Shih-Chen, L. 1578. Ben cao or *Pen Ts'ao*).

Sole, J.D. et al. 1983. The vascular flora of Lilley Cornett Woods, Letcher County, Kentucky. *Castanea*. 48: 174-88.

Staba, E.J. and S.E. Chen. 1979. An Overview of Ginseng Chemistry, Pharmacology and Anti-Tumor Effects. *Proc. 1st Nat. Ginseng Conf.*, Lexington, KY 91-100; quoted in Duke, J.A., op. cit., p. 119.

Strombom, J. 1985. Studies on absorption and distribution of ginsenoside Rg1 by whole-body autoradiography and chromatography. *Acta Pharm. Suec*. 22: 113-22.

Takaku, T. et al. 1990. Studies on insulin-like substances in Korean red ginseng. *Planta Medica* 56: 27-30.

Tang, W. and G. Eisenbrand. 1992. *Chinese Drugs of Plant Origin*. New York: Springer-Verlag.

Teeguarden, R. 1984. *Chinese Tonic Herbs*. New York: Japan Publications.

Thompson, G.A. 1991 (1987). Botanical Characteristics of Ginseng. *Herbs, Spices, and Medicinal Plants,* vol. 2, pp. 111-36. Binghamton, NY: Haworth Press, Inc.

Tode, T. 1993. Inhibitory effects by oral administration of ginsenoside Rh2 on the growth of human ovarian cancer cells in nude mice. *J. Cancer Res. Clin. Oncol.:* 120: 24-26.

Tomoda, M. et al. 1993. Characterization of two novel polysaccharides having immunological activities from the root of Panax ginseng. *Biological and Pharmaceutical Bulletin* 16:1087-90.

Tu, G. (Ed. In Chief). 1988. *Pharmacopeia of the People's Republic of China* (English Edition 1988). Beijing: People's Medical Publishing House.

Turner, C. 1995. Canada discovers a root to wealth. *LA Times* 114 (Sat., Oct. 7): D1, col 2.

Vogel, V. 1970. *American Indian Medicine.* Norman: University of Oklahoma Press.

Von Ardenne, M. 1987. Measurements of the increase in the difference between the arterial and venous Hb-oxygen saturation obtained with daily administration of 200 mg standardized ginseng extract G115 for four weeks: Long-term increase of the oxygen transport into the organs and tissues of the organism through biologically active substances. *Panminerva Medica.* 29: 143-50.

Waller, D.P. et al. 1992. Lack of Androgenicity of Siberian Ginseng. letter, *JAMA;* 267: 2329.

Walters, C. 1995. Restoring Ginseng's Vital Force. *Acres, U.S.A.* June.

Wang, J. 1982. Quantitative determination of saponins in the roots of Panax notoginseng, P. ginseng and P. quinquefolius. *Yaozue Tongbao.* 17: 244-45.

Wang, S. and G. Zhu. 1990. Effects of Codonopsis pilosulae on the synthesis of thromboxane A2 and prostacyclin. *Chung Hsi I Chieh Ho Tsa Chih.* 10(7): 391-94, 387

Wang, Y. L. et al. 1994. Effects and mechanism of total saponins of Panax Notoginseng on anti- inflammation and analgesia. *Chung Kuo Chung Hsi I Chieh Ho Tsa Chih.* 14: 35-36, 5-6.

Watanabe, H. et al. 1991. Effect of Panax ginseng on age-related changes in the spontaneous motor activity and dopaminergic system in the rat. *Japanese Journal of Pharmacology.* 55: 51-56.

Wei, J. and R. An. 1983. Determination of trace elements in Panax ginseng C.A. Meyer from Jilin. (China). *Baichiuen Yike Daxue Xuebao* 9: 58-59.

Wolfe, T. 1995. An ecological success story: The Wisconsin Ginseng Project. *Pathways* (Summer), pp. 35ff.

Wong, C.K. et al. 1994. The induction of cytokine gene expression in murine peritoneal macrophages by Pseudostellaria heterophylla. *Immunopharmacol Immunotoxicol.* 16: 347-57.

Wu, Q.F. et al. 1991. Purification and identification of red ginseng polypeptides. *Yao Hsueh Hsueh Pao* 26: 499-504.

Yamamoto, M. 1983. Serum HDL-cholesterol-increasing and fatty liver-improving actions of Panax ginseng in high cholesterol diet-fed rats with clinical effect on hyperlipidemia in man. *Am. J. Chin. Med.* 1: 96-101.

Yun, T.K. & S.Y. Choi. 1990. A case-control study of ginseng intake and cancer. *Int. J. Epidemiol.* 19: 871-86.

Yun, T.K. and S.Y. Choi. 1995. Preventive effect of ginseng intake against various human cancers: a case-control study on 1987 pairs. *Cancer Epidemiol. Biomarkers Prev.* 4: 401-08.

Zhan, Y. et al. 1994. Protective effects of ginsenoside on myocardiac ischemic and reperfusion injuries. *Chung Hua I Hsueh Tsa Chih* 74: 626-28, 648.

Zhang, Y. 1983. Different processings of ginseng and saponin content in different parts of plant for medical use. *Zhongcaoyao.* 14: 211-12.

Zhao, X.Z. 1990. Antisenility effect of ginseng-rhizome saponin. *Chung Hsi I Chieh Ho Tsa Chih* 10: 586-89, 579.

Zneg, X.L. et al. 1992. Immunological and hematopoietic effect of Codonopsis pilosula on cancer patients during radiotherapy. *Chung Kuo Chung Hsi I Chieh Ho Tsa Chih* 1992; 12: 607-08, 581

Zuin, M. 1987. Effects of a preparation containing a standardized ginseng extract combined with trace elements and multivitamins against hepatotoxin-induced chronic liver disease in the elderly. *J. Int. Med. Res.* 15: 276-81.

— NOTES —